In memory of
Sir Richard Doll (1912–2005) and Ruth Roemer (1916–2005)
for their lifetime achievements in battling the tobacco pandemic.

Also published by the
American Cancer Society:

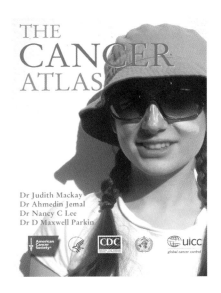

THE
CANCER
ATLAS

Dr Judith Mackay
Dr Ahmedin Jemal
Dr Nancy C Lee
Dr D Maxwell Parkin

THE TOBACCO ATLAS

SECOND EDITION

Dr Judith Mackay
Dr Michael Eriksen
Dr Omar Shafey

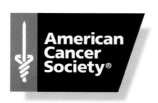

Published by the American Cancer Society
1599 Clifton Road NE
Atlanta, Georgia 30329, USA
www.cancer.org

1 3 5 7 9 10 8 6 4 2

ISBN 0-944235-58-1

Library of Congress Cataloging-in-Publication Data
Mackay, Judith. *The Tobacco Atlas* / Dr Judith Mackay, Dr Michael Eriksen,
Dr Omar Shafey. 2nd ed.
p. cm.
Includes bibliographical references and index.
ISBN 0-944235-58-1 (paperback)
1. Tobacco use-Maps. 2. Tobacco industry-Maps. 3. Medical geography.
I. Eriksen, Michael P. II. Shafey, Omar. III. American Cancer Society. IV. Title.
G1046.J94M3 2006
362.29'60223-dc22
2005045006

Produced for the American Cancer Society by
Myriad Editions Limited
6–7 Old Steine, Brighton BN1 1EJ, UK
www.MyriadEditions.com

Edited and co-ordinated for Myriad Editions by
Candida Lacey, Jannet King and Sadie Mayne
Design and graphics by Corinne Pearlman and Isabelle Lewis
Maps created by Isabelle Lewis

Printed on paper produced from sustainable sources.
Printed and bound in Hong Kong through Phoenix Offset Limited
under the supervision of Bob Cassels, The Hanway Press, London

CONTENTS

Reviews of the first edition of *The Tobacco Atlas*:

"*The Tobacco Atlas* is the best thing of its
kind I've ever seen."
— C Everett Koop, former US Surgeon General

"Informative, so easy to read, beautiful to look at."
— Annie J Sasco
International Agency for Research on Cancer

"I love the atlas! A gold-mine."
— Ruben Israel
GLOBALink

"It's really helpful and an informative guide for tobacco
control advocates."
— Syed Mahbubul Alam Tahin
Work for a Better Bangladesh

"A comprehensive, attractively produced profile of all major
aspects of the tobacco epidemic and what has been
done so far to try to reduce it."
— David Simpson
International Agency on Tobacco and Health

"A manual of immense value for all people involved
in smoking control."
— Kjell Bjartveit
Norway

"A beautiful and informative book."
— Tai Hing Lam
Department of Community Medicine
University of Hong Kong

"*The Tobacco Atlas* is excellent."
— Gérard Dubois
Service d'Evaluation Médicale, France

"A definite hit."
— Judy Wilkenfeld
Campaign for Tobacco-Free Kids, USA

FOREWORD

A message from

John R Seffrin, PhD
Chief Executive Officer
American Cancer Society

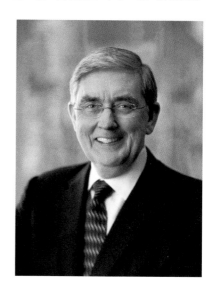

Whithat if the world, and especially its developing nations, were under sustained, strategic assault from a powerful entity with nefarious motives? What if our children – all of them – were a particular target of this evil entity? That is precisely what is happening in the world today, and the assaulting entity is neither an individual nor a nation. Instead, the world is facing a pandemic of epic proportions because it is under attack by a ruthless industry – the purveyors of tobacco. Employing insidious and immoral marketing tactics to lure the world's youth into a life of addiction and disease, the tobacco industry is a plague that generates suffering on a par with the ravages of war, famine, and poverty. It is incumbent on the citizens of the world to unite and extinguish the tobacco threat to save future generations from the predations of this death-dealing juggernaut.

Tobacco, the only consumer product proven to kill more than half of its regular users, is responsible for about 5 million deaths worldwide every year. Today, that burden is roughly evenly divided between industrialized and developing nations. However, if current trends continue through 2025, tobacco will kill 10 million people worldwide each and every year and 7 million of these deaths will be in the developing world, in nations least prepared to deal with the financial, social, and political consequences of this global public health tragedy.

If we fail to act to prevent this tragedy, the consequences will most certainly be dire. Tobacco will eventually kill about 650 million smokers alive today, about 10% of the current total world population. Half of these people will die in middle age – when they are most productive for their economies, their societies, and their families. In

the last century alone, tobacco killed 100 million smokers. If left unchecked, tobacco will kill more than 1 billion people in this century.

This extraordinary suffering and death is not inevitable, however. Without intervention, the tobacco pandemic will be the worst case of avoidable loss of life in recorded history. Yet, with comprehensive, concerted action, we can eliminate the global scourge of tobacco and save hundreds of millions of lives within the next few decades.

How can we do it? We must help current smokers quit and prevent the tobacco industry from using its reprehensible marketing techniques to lure more of the world's children into deadly addiction. If we choose to act, the number of lives saved could be astronomical. For example, if we were able to cut adult cigarette consumption by just 50 percent worldwide, we could avert more than 300 million needless deaths within the next 50 years. That's 300 million real people – mothers and fathers, children and siblings – people who enrich their cultures, people who sustain their economies, and people who are loved by their families.

As smoking rates decline in the USA and many other industrialized nations, the tobacco industry has dramatically stepped up its efforts in the emerging markets of Asia, Africa, and Latin America. Because tobacco kills its long-term customers, the industry must cultivate millions of new smokers each year just to break even. In the less restricted markets of the developing world, that means that no one is immune from the industry's tactics, especially the most vulnerable people of all – children.

Today, worldwide, one in seven teenagers aged 13 to 15 smokes. One-quarter of them tried their first cigarette before the age of 10. Nearly 100,000 children and adolescents become addicted worldwide *every day*. And it's no wonder. In the USA alone, the tobacco industry spent $15.15 billion in 2003 to market its products; that's more than $1.7 million every hour of every day.

Fortunately, thanks to the rigorous educational, scientific, and advocacy efforts of dedicated tobacco control activists worldwide, many nations of the world are taking a stand against tobacco by supporting the world's first global public health treaty – the World Health Organization's Framework Convention on Tobacco Control (FCTC). In fact, the campaign to reduce the global burden of tobacco-related disease celebrated a significant victory in November 2004 with the FCTC's ratification, a tremendous milestone for global public health. Now the challenge is to implement and enforce the FCTC's provisions so that we can save millions of lives each year just by reducing tobacco consumption.

Now, with the publication of this revised and updated second edition of *The Tobacco Atlas*, we take another important step forward in our collective efforts. This timely, evidence-based publication offers a wealth of compelling data to help tobacco control advocates of every nation combat the menace of tobacco in their communities, their nations, and the world. Information is a powerful tool in the hands of passionate, dedicated individuals, and this book provides an unparalleled resource to arm and inform tobacco's opponents worldwide.

In addition to the leading-edge data we need to inform our tobacco control strategies, *The Tobacco Atlas* also provides a more intangible, but no less powerful, weapon – hope. For the significant updates and exciting developments chronicled in this publication prove that we are indeed making progress against tobacco. Our broad network of determined activists is achieving positive change at the local, national, and international levels. Together, we are empowering the world to defend itself against the tobacco industry's relentless assault. With *The Tobacco Atlas* in our arsenal, we will continue to move toward victory over tobacco.

JOHN R SEFFRIN
Atlanta, USA

PREFACE

This book is intended for anyone concerned with personal or political health, governance, politics, economics, big business, corporate behaviour, globalization, smuggling, tax, religion, the internet, allocation of resources, poverty, gender issues, human rights, children, human development and the future.

This second edition of *The Tobacco Atlas* maps the history and current situation, and makes some predictions for the future of the tobacco epidemic up to the year 2050. It illustrates how tobacco is not just a simple health issue, but involves the whole of government, economics, big business, politics, trade, crimes such as smuggling, litigation and deceit.

The atlas also shows the importance of a multifaceted approach to reducing the epidemic, by WHO, other UN agencies, non-governmental organizations (NGOs), the private and business sector – in fact, the whole of civil society.

Since the first edition of *The Tobacco Atlas* was published in 2002, there have been several significant developments in tobacco control. The main one is the WHO Framework Convention on Tobacco Control (FCTC), which came into effect in 2005, and which uniquely uses international law to further public health.

One valuable extension of making the data more available has been the creation of an interactive, online version of this atlas, available at http://www.tobaccoresearch.net/atlas.html. In addition, more research has been undertaken, especially in developing countries. The economics of tobacco has been more carefully studied, showing that tobacco control is good for the wealth as well as the health of nations. More countries have passed legislation such as bans on tobacco promotion, the requirement of health warnings, and the creation of smoke-free areas in public places, while other countries have increased taxation, expanded national capacity and analyzed tobacco industry documents, exposing the activities of the tobacco industry in their country. Bhutan has become the first country in the world to ban tobacco sales.

Yet, despite this progress and mostly due to population increases in the world, the number of smokers and the number of tobacco-related deaths is rising. This unfortunate trend is likely to continue for the foreseeable future. This burden is falling increasingly on developing countries, and the concern that more women are smoking cannot be underestimated.

The publication of this second edition marks a critical juncture in the epidemic. We stand at a crossroads, with the future in our hands. We can choose to stand aside or take weak and ineffective measures. Alternatively we can embrace the spirit and letter of the Framework Convention on Tobacco Control and implement robust and enduring measures to protect the health and wealth of nations. History will judge the course taken and the outcome will be measured in millions of lives.

JUDITH MACKAY
Asian Consultancy on Tobacco Control
Hong Kong SAR, China

MICHAEL ERIKSEN
Georgia State University
Atlanta, USA

OMAR SHAFEY
American Cancer Society
Atlanta, USA

ACKNOWLEDGEMENTS

Sincere thanks to the American Cancer Society, the Georgia Cancer Coalition and the Western Pacific Regional Office of the World Health Organization for their generous financial support of the second edition of *The Tobacco Atlas*.

An interactive, online version of this atlas is available at the Global Tobacco Research Network site: http://www.tobaccoresearch.net/atlas.html and we are grateful to the Johns Hopkins Bloomberg School of Public Health's Institute for Global Tobacco Control, the American Cancer Society and the National Cancer Institute, for supporting this site, which has been developed by Myriad Editions.

Many people have helped in the preparation of this atlas. First, we especially would like to thank our principal researchers: Priti Bandi, Department of Epidemiology and Surveillance Research, American Cancer Society, USA; David Boisclair, Health Economist, Montreal, Canada; Valerie Bycott, Institute of Public Health, Georgia State University, USA; Stacy Crim, Department of Epidemiology and Surveillance Research, American Cancer Society, USA; G Emmanuel Guindon, Department of Research Policy and Cooperation, World Health Organization; Anna Jeanne Layton, International Affairs Department, American Cancer Society, USA; and Stacey Martin, Institute of Public Health, Georgia State University, USA.

The headquarters and regional offices of the World Health Organization cooperated fully in the production of this edition, and we would also like to acknowledge their support for the first edition.

The International Union Against Cancer (UICC) supplied much information, for which we are grateful.

For their advice on particular maps and subjects, we would like to thank the following individuals:

1 Types of tobacco use
Samira Asma, Office on Smoking and Health, Centers for Disease Control and Prevention, USA; Prakash Gupta, Healis Sekhsaria Institute of Public Health, Mumbai, India.

2 Male smoking and **3 Female smoking**
Kate Strong, Acting Team Leader, WHO Global InfoBase (GIF).

5 Boys' tobacco use and **6 Girls' tobacco use**
Cheryll J Cardinez, Cancer Surveillance Branch, Division of Cancer Prevention and Control, Centers for Disease Control and Prevention, USA; Wick Warren, Office on Smoking and Health, Centers for Disease Control and Prevention, USA; Samira Asma, Office on Smoking and Health, Centers for Disease Control and Prevention, USA; Nancy C Lee, Consultant, Division of Cancer Prevention and Control, Centers for Disease Control and Prevention, USA.

8 Health risks
Michael Thun, Department of Epidemiology and Surveillance Research, American Cancer Society, USA; Elizabeth Ward, Department of Epidemiology and Surveillance Research, American Cancer Society, USA.

10 Deaths
Majid Ezzati, Department of Population and International Health, Harvard School of Public Health, USA; Teh-wei Hu, University of California, Berkeley, USA.

11 Costs to the economy
Steven Tobin, Organization for Economic Co-operation and Development (OECD).

12 Costs to the smoker
Gbenga Adejuwoon, Tobacco Free Youth, Nigeria; Natalia Alexeeva, Institute of Internal Medicine, Russian Federation; Susan Asiimwe, The Environmental Action Network, Uganda; Kamel Bereksi, Polyclinique Jean Kraft, Algeria; Hatai Chitanondh, The National Health Foundation, Thailand; Andjelka Dzeletovic, Institute of Public Health of Serbia, Serbia & Montenegro; Tim Frasca, Fundacion Cipress, Chile; Muna Hamzeh, Ministry of Health, Jordan; Charles Kassa, Pontentiel 2000 ONG, Benin; Outhaki Khamphoui, Gender Resource Information and Development Center, Laos; Andranik Melikjanyan, Lore Eco Club NGO, Armenia; Adriana Menéndez, Sindicato Medico del Uruguay,

Uruguay; Manjari Peiris, journalist, Sri Lanka; Tibor Szilágyi, Health 21 Hungarian Foundation, Hungary; Anna White, Global Partnerships for Tobacco Control, Essential Action, USA.

15 Tobacco companies
Samira Asma, Office on Smoking and Health, Centers for Disease Control and Prevention, USA.

17 Illegal cigarettes
Luk Joossens, International Union Against Cancer (UICC); Eric LeGresley, tobacco control consultant, Canada.

18 Marketing
Samira Asma, Office on Smoking and Health, Centers for Disease Control and Prevention, USA; Stanton Glantz, Center for Tobacco Control Research and Education, University of California, San Francisco, USA; Amei Zhang and Darryl Jayson, Tobacco Merchants Association, USA.

21 Research
Rosemary Kennedy, Research for International Tobacco Control (RITC), International Development Research Centre, Canada; Carrie J Matson, Institute for Global Tobacco Control (IGTC), Johns Hopkins Bloomberg School of Public Health, USA; Hana Ross, RTI International, Research Triangle Institute, USA; Frances Stillman, Institute for Global Tobacco Control (IGTC), Johns Hopkins Bloomberg School of Public Health, USA; Linda Waverly, International Development Research Centre (IDRC), Canada; Derek Yach, Community Action to Prevent Chronic Disease (CAPCoD), Yale School of Public Health, USA.

22 Capacity building
Bjarne Rosted, International Affairs, Norwegian Cancer Society, Norway; Laurent Huber, Framework Convention Alliance for Tobacco Control.

23 Framework Convention on Tobacco Control
Douglas Bettcher, Tobacco Free Initiative, World Health Organization.

24 Smoke-free areas
Ana Navas-Acien, Department of Epidemiology, Johns Hopkins Bloomberg School of Public Health, USA.

26 Warning labels
Hatai Chitanondh, The National Health Foundation, Thailand; Geoffrey Fong, Department of Psychology, University of Waterloo, Canada.

27 Health education
Marjo Pyykönen, International Quit & Win, Finland.

29 Tobacco tax
Anne-Marie Perucic, Tobacco Free Initiative, World Health Organization.

30 Litigation
Richard A Daynard, Northeastern University School of Law, USA; Mark Gottlieb, Tobacco Control Resource Center, Tobacco Products Liability Project, USA; Edward L Sweda, Jr, Tobacco Control Resource Center, Tobacco Products Liability Project, USA.

31 The future
Colin Mathers, Evidence and Information for Policy, World Health Organization.

The history of tobacco
John Bickerstaff, International Network Towards SmokeFree Hospitals, UK; Gene Borio, Tobacco News and Information; Simon Chapman, *Tobacco Control*; Joe Cherner, SmokeFree Educational Services, Inc; Sheila Duffy, Information and Communications, ASH Scotland; Margaretha Haglund, National Institute of Public Health, Sweden; Hong-Gwan Seo, National Cancer Center, Republic of Korea; Ruben Israel, GLOBALink; Sinéad Jones, Tobacco Control, International Union Against Cancer (UICC); Michael Tacelosky, SmokeFree Educational Services, Inc.

For their diverse talents and editorial expertise, and individual as well as collective contributions, we would like to thank the team at Myriad Editions: Candida Lacey, Jannet King, Corinne Pearlman, Isabelle Lewis and Sadie Mayne.

Finally, we want to thank our families for their support during the preparation of this atlas.

PHOTO CREDITS

ABOUT THE AUTHORS

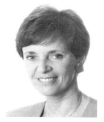

Dr Judith Mackay is a medical doctor based in Hong Kong. She is a Senior Policy Advisor to the World Health Organization, and holds professorships at the Chinese Academy of Preventive Medicine in Beijing, and the Department of Community Medicine at the University of Hong Kong. After an early career as a hospital physician, she moved to working in preventive and public health. She is a Fellow of the Royal Colleges of Physicians of Edinburgh and of London. Dr Mackay has received many international awards, including the WHO Commemorative Medal, a Royal Award from the King of Thailand, the Fries Prize for Improving Health, the Luther Terry Award for Outstanding Individual Leadership, the International Partnering for World Health Award, and the Founding International Achievement Award from the Asia Pacific Association for the Control of Tobacco. She co-authored the first edition of *The Tobacco Atlas* and is the author of several other Myriad atlases, including *The State of Health Atlas*, *The Penguin Atlas of Human Sexual Behavior*, *The Atlas of Heart Disease and Stroke* and *The Cancer Atlas*.

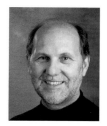

Dr Michael Eriksen is Professor and founding Director of the Institute of Public Health at Georgia State University. Prior to his current position, Dr Eriksen served as a Senior Advisor to the World Health Organization in Geneva and was Director of CDC's Office on Smoking and Health, serving in this capacity from 1992 to 2000. Dr Eriksen has published extensively on tobacco prevention and control and has served as an expert witness in litigation against the tobacco industry. He is Editor-in-Chief of *Health Education Research* and has been designated as a Distinguished Cancer Scholar by the Georgia Cancer Coalition. He is a recipient of the WHO Commemorative Medal on Tobacco or Health and a Presidential Citation for Meritorious Service by former President Clinton. He is Past President and Distinguished Fellow of the Society for Public Health Education and, for 30 years, he has been a member of the American Public Health Association.

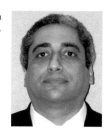

Dr Omar Shafey, a medical anthropologist and epidemiologist, manages the American Cancer Society's International Tobacco Surveillance program. He is an adjunct professor in the Global Health Department of the Rollins School of Public Health at Emory University in Atlanta, Georgia, USA. He edited the *Tobacco Control Country Profiles 2003* and has published research articles on smoking among women in Spain, cigarette smuggling in Brazil, and lung cancer trends among young adults in the USA.

GLOSSARY

Information about different types of tobacco use is given on pp18–19.

Addiction – Physiological or psychological dependence on a substance characterized by neurochemical changes, compulsive drug-seeking behaviour, dose tolerance, withdrawal symptoms, uncontrolled craving, and self-destructive behaviour. Common addictive drugs include alcohol, opiates, and nicotine.

Advertising – Any form of commercial communication, recommendation or action with the aim of promoting a tobacco product or tobacco use, either directly or indirectly, including point-of-sale, direct mail, magazine, newspaper, or outdoor advertising. Includes sponsorship.

BCE – Before the Common Era.

Bupropion – an antidepressant pharmaceutical used to help people quit smoking.

Cancer – A type of disease in which abnormal cells divide uncontrollably. Cancer cells can invade nearby tissues and spread through the bloodstream and lymphatic system to other parts of the body. Tobacco consumption significantly increases the risk of developing many types of cancers.

Carcinogen – A substance that causes cancer. Tobacco contains many potent chemical carcinogens, including tobacco-specific nitrosamines (TSNs), polyaromatic hydrocarbons (PAHs), and volatile organic compounds (VOCs).

Chronic bronchitis – Inflammation of the bronchial mucous membrane characterized by cough, hypersecretion of mucus, and expectoration of sputum over a long period of time, associated with increased vulnerability to bronchial infection. *See also* Chronic obstructive pulmonary disease.

Chronic obstructive pulmonary disease (COPD) – A chronic lung disease, such as asthma or emphysema, in which breathing becomes slowed or forced. *See also* Chronic bronchitis.

Consumption – Total cigarette consumption is the number of cigarettes sold annually in a country, usually in millions of sticks. Total cigarette consumption is calculated by adding a country's cigarette production and imports and subtracting exports. "Per adult" cigarette consumption is calculated by dividing total cigarette consumption by the total population of those who are 15 years and older. Smuggling may account for inaccuracies in these estimates.

Coronary artery disease/coronary heart disease – The narrowing or blockage of the coronary arteries (blood vessels that carry blood and oxygen to the heart) usually caused by atherosclerosis (a build up of fatty material and plaque inside the coronary arteries).

Costs – Macroeconomic costs associated with tobacco use. *Direct costs*: health costs related to diseases caused by tobacco; health-service costs, such as hospital services, physician and outpatient services, prescription drugs, nursing-home services, home healthcare, allied healthcare; changed expenditures due to increased utilization of services.

Indirect costs: productivity costs caused by tobacco-related illness or premature death; loss of productivity and earnings.
Total costs: The sum of direct and indirect tobacco-attributable costs to society.

Cotinine – Nicotine's major metabolite, which has a significantly longer half-life than nicotine. Cotinine measurement is often used to estimate a patient's tobacco/nicotine usage prior to quitting, and to confirm abstinence self-reports during follow-up. Cotinine is commonly measured in serum, urine, and saliva.

Emphysema – A pathological condition of the lungs marked by an abnormal increase in the size of the air spaces, resulting in laboured breathing and an increased susceptibility to infection. It can be caused by irreversible expansion of the alveoli, or by the destruction of alveolar walls.

Environmental tobacco smoke (ETS) – Smoke inhaled by an individual not actively engaged in smoking. It contains the same harmful chemicals that smokers inhale. *See also* Passive smoking.

Excess mortality – The amount by which death rates for a given population group (eg smokers) exceed that of another population group chosen as a reference or standard (eg non-smokers).

Framework Convention on Tobacco Control – The WHO Framework Convention on Tobacco Control (WHO FCTC) is the first treaty negotiated under the auspices of the World Health Organization. It lays down an international, legal template for action on tobacco control.

Global Youth Tobacco Survey (GYTS) – The World Health Organization (WHO) and Centers for Disease Control and Prevention (CDC) developed the GYTS to track tobacco use among young people across countries, using a common methodology and core questionnaire.

Health professionals – Includes, in the context of this atlas: anaesthetists, clinical nurses, dental students (third-year), dentists, health-science students, hospital staff, medical doctors, medical residents, medical students (pre-clinical, clinical-year and third-year), nursing students, pharmacy students (third-year).

Health warnings – Verbal, written or visual warnings, required by governments on packets or advertisements of all tobacco products.

Ingredient – Every component of the product that is smoked or chewed, including all additives and flavourings, contents such as paper, ink and filters, and materials used in the manufacturing process (such as adhesives etc) present in the finished product in burnt or unburned form.

Marketing – A range of activities aimed at ensuring continued sales and profitability of a product. These include advertising, promotions, public relations and sales.

Nicotiana tabacum – The tobacco plant. Its leaves contain high levels of the addictive chemical nicotine and many cancer-causing chemicals. The leaves may be smoked (in cigarettes, cigars, and pipes), applied to the gums (as dipping and chewing tobacco), or inhaled (as snuff). Tobacco use and exposure to secondhand tobacco smoke causes many types of cancer, as well as heart, respiratory, and other diseases.

Nicotine – An addictive, poisonous alkaloid chemical found in tobacco that acts as a stimulant, increasing heart rate and use of oxygen by cardiac muscle. Also used as an insecticide. The lethal dose for a human adult is about 50mg.

Nicotine replacement therapy (NRT) – A type of treatment for smoking that aids cessation by providing a low dose of nicotine to ease cravings experienced by addicted smokers. NRTs include devices such as transdermal patches, nicotine gum, nicotine nasal sprays and inhalers.

Passive smoking – Inhaling cigarette, cigar, or pipe smoke produced by another individual. It is composed of second-hand smoke (exhaled by the smoker), and sidestream smoke (which drifts off the tip of the cigarette or cigar or pipe bowl). Also known as environmental tobacco smoke (ETS).

Polyaromatic hydrocarbon (PAH) – A type of organic compound composed of several benzene rings. PAHs, many of which are carcinogenic, are produced during charbroiling of meat, incomplete combustion of fossil fuels, and burning of tobacco. Tobacco smoke is the most important source of human exposure.

Prevalence – Smoking prevalence is the percentage of smokers in the total population. Adult smoking is usually defined as smoking among those aged 15 years and older.

Promotion – Includes special offers, gifts, price discounts, coupons, company websites, speciality item distribution and telephone advertising used to facilitate the sale or placement of any cigarette. Also includes allowances paid to cigarette retailers, wholesalers, full-time company employees or any other persons involved in cigarette distribution.

Retailer – A person engaged in a business that includes the sale of a tobacco product to consumers.

Risk – The likelihood of incurring a particular event or circumstance (eg risk of disease measures the chances of an individual contracting a disease).

Smoke-free area – Area where smoking or holding a lighted cigarette, cigar or pipe is banned.

Smokeless tobacco – Includes snuff and chewing tobacco; not a safe alternative to smoking. Smokeless tobacco is as addictive as smoking and can cause cancer of the gum, cheek, lip, mouth, tongue, and throat.

Smoker – Someone who, at the time of the survey, smokes any tobacco product either daily or occasionally.

Stroke – A condition in which a blood vessel in the brain bursts or is clogged by a blood clot. This leads to an inadequate blood supply to the brain and death of the brain cells, and usually results in temporary or permanent neurological deficits.

Tar – The raw anhydrous nicotine-free condensate of smoke.

Tar and nicotine yield – The amount of tar and nicotine in milligrammes in one cigarette, as determined by a machine designed to measure smoke. Machine yields of tar and nicotine levels are not necessarily what smokers actually inhale.

Tobacco-attributable mortality – The number of deaths attributable to tobacco use within a specific population.

Tobacco control organization – A non-profit organization, the purpose of which is to reduce tobacco consumption and protect nonsmokers from the effects of involuntary smoking.

Tobacco industry documents – Previously secret, internal industry papers that have now been placed in the public domain as a result of court rulings.

Tobacco product – Any product manufactured wholly or partly from tobacco and intended for use by smoking, inhalation, chewing, sniffing or sucking, with the exception of medicinal preparations containing nicotine.

Tobacco production – Tobacco-leaf production in metric tonnes refers to the actual tobacco leaves harvested from the field, excluding harvesting and threshing losses and any part of the tobacco crop not harvested for any reason.

Tobacco-specific nitrosamine (TSN or TSNA) – A group of seven toxic chemicals found only in tobacco products. N'-nitrosonornicotine (NNN), (4-methylnitrosamino)-1-(3-pyridyl)-1-butanone (NNK), and N-oxide, 4-(methylnitrosamino)-1-(3-pyridyl N-oxide)-1-butanol (NNAL; a metabolic product of NNK), are the most carcinogenic.

Tobacco taxes – The sum of all types of taxes levied on tobacco products. There are two basic methods of tobacco taxation:
Nominal or specific taxes: based on a set amount of tax per unit (eg cigarette) or gramme of tobacco. These taxes are often differentiated according to the type of tobacco product (eg filtered *vs* non-filtered cigarettes, pipe tobacco *vs* cigars).
Ad valorem taxes: assessed as a percentage markup on some determined value (tax base), usually the retail selling price of tobacco products or a wholesale price. These taxes include any value-added tax (VAT) where applicable.

Tobacco use – The consumption of tobacco products by burning, chewing, inhalation, or other forms of ingestion.

Volatile organic compound (VOC) – An organic (carbon-containing) compound that evaporates at room temperature. VOCs contribute significantly to indoor air pollution and respiratory disease.

Warning labels – Verbal, written or visual warnings, required by governments on packets or advertisements of all tobacco products. *See also* Health warnings.

1 Types of tobacco use

Cigarettes account for the largest share of manufactured tobacco products in the world – 96 percent of total sales. Except for chewing tobacco in India and possibly kreteks in Indonesia, cigarettes are the most common method of consuming tobacco throughout the world.

The invention of the cigarette-rolling machine in 1881 accelerated the tobacco pandemic by mass-producing pocket-sized packets of cigarettes. Unlike tediously hand-rolled cigarettes and bulky water pipes, manufactured cigarettes offered a convenient and portable method to maintain addiction, even while driving a motor vehicle, working in an factory, or watching a movie.

In the current era of economic globalization, some forms of tobacco, historically localized to specific regions of the world (such as the hookah and bidi), have spread far beyond the Middle East and South Asia to every continent. For instance, Indonesian kreteks, clove-flavoured, loosely packed tobacco cigarettes, are currently being marketed to youth in many industrialized countries. These regional forms of tobacco sometimes gain footholds in new countries based on their exotic cachet but they rarely, if ever, displace manufactured cigarettes for a significant market share. Instead, they frequently serve as a gateway to addiction, luring youth and other fad smokers into a lifelong dependence on cigarettes.

Manufactured cigarettes

Manufactured cigarettes consist of shredded or reconstituted tobacco, processed with hundreds of chemicals. Often tipped with a filter, they are manufactured by a machine, and are now the predominant manner in which tobacco is consumed worldwide.

Cigarettes are available throughout the world. Filter-tipped cigarettes are usually more popular than unfiltered cigarettes.

Roll-your-own (RYO) cigarettes

Roll-your-own cigarettes are hand-filled cigarettes made by the smoker from fine-cut, loose tobacco and a cigarette paper.

Sometimes a small hand-held rolling machine is used. RYO cigarettes contain the same toxic and carcinogenic constituents as manufactured cigarettes. RYO cigarette smokers are exposed to high concentrations of tobacco particulates, tar, nicotine and tobacco-specific nitrosamines (TSNAs) and they experience increased risks for cancers of the mouth, pharynx, larynx, lung and oesophagus.

Moist snuff

A small amount of ground tobacco is held in the mouth between the cheek and gum. Increasingly manufacturers are pre-packaging moist snuff into small paper or cloth packets, to make the product easier to use. Other smokeless tobacco products include khaini, shammaah, nass or naswa.

Cigars

Cigars are made of air-cured and fermented tobaccos with a tobacco-leaf wrapper, and come in many shapes and sizes, from cigarette-sized cigarillos, double coronas, cheroots, stumpen, chuttas and dhumtis. In reverse chutta and dhumti smoking, the ignited end of the cigar is placed inside the mouth. There has been a revival of cigar-smoking since the end of the 20th century among both men and women.

There is no safe way of using tobacco – whether it is inhaled, sniffed, sucked, chewed, or mixed with other ingredients.

Bidis

Bidis consist of a small amount of tobacco, hand-wrapped in dried temburni or tendu leaf and tied with string. Despite their small size, their tar and carbon monoxide deliveries can be higher than manufactured cigarettes because of the need to puff harder to keep bidis lit.

Bidis are found throughout South Asia, and are India's most used type of tobacco.

Water pipes

The water pipe, also known as shisha, hookah or hubble-bubble, is commonly used in North Africa, the Mediterranean region and parts of Asia.

Sticks

Sticks are made from sun-cured tobacco and wrapped in cigarette paper, for example, hand-rolled brus, popular in Papua New Guinea.

Chewing tobacco

Chewing tobacco is also known as plug, loose-leaf, chimo, toombak, gutkha and twist. Pan masala or betel quid consists of tobacco, areca nuts and slaked lime wrapped in a betel leaf. They can also contain sweetenings and flavouring agents. Varieties of pan include kaddipudi, hogesoppu, gundi, kadapam, zarda, pattiwala, kiwam and mishri.

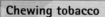

Tobacco is used orally throughout the world, but principally in South-East Asia. In Mumbai, India, 56% of women chew tobacco.

Kreteks

Kreteks are clove-flavoured cigarettes widely smoked in Indonesia. They may also contain a wide range of exotic flavourings and eugenol, which has an anesthetic effect, allowing for greater and deeper inhalation.

Pipes

Pipes are made of briar, slate, clay or other substance. Tobacco is placed in the bowl and the smoke is inhaled through the stem.

In South-East Asia, clay pipes known as suipa, chilum, and hookli are widely used.

Dry snuff

Dry snuff is powdered tobacco that is inhaled through the nose or taken orally. Once widespread, its use is now in decline.

19

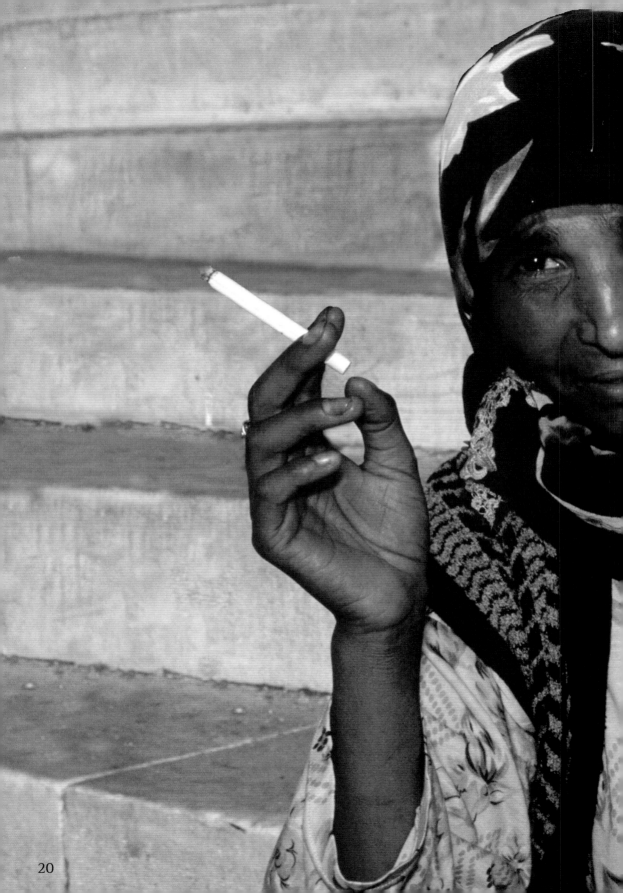

PART ONE

PREVALENCE AND HEALTH

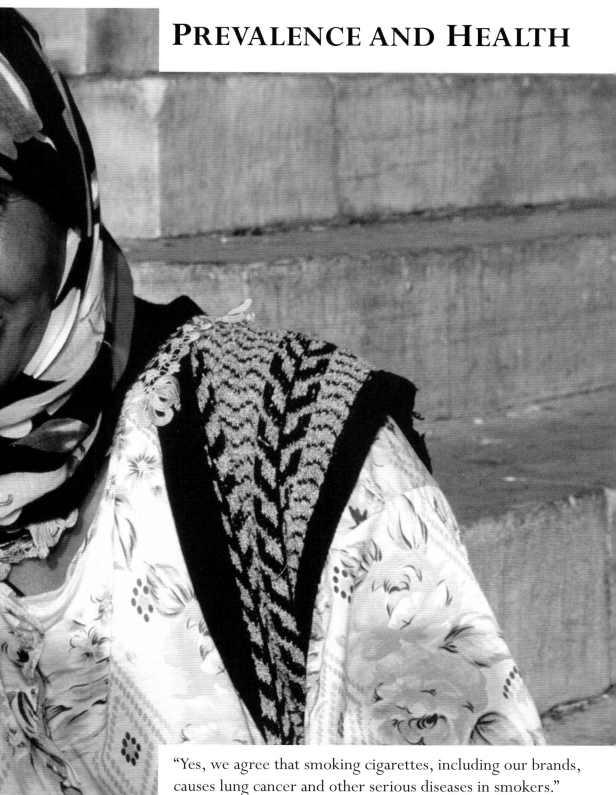

"Yes, we agree that smoking cigarettes, including our brands, causes lung cancer and other serious diseases in smokers."

Thomas Dubois, Director, Corporate Affairs, Philip Morris Australia, 2002

Male smoking

"Life is too precious, do not destroy it."
Mother Teresa (1910–97)

Smoking has been portrayed by its sellers as a masculine habit, linked to health, happiness, fitness, wealth, power, and sexual success. In reality, it leads to sickness, premature death, sexual impotence and infertility.

Almost 1 billion men in the world smoke – about 35 percent of men in developed countries, and 50 percent of men in developing countries. Trends in both developed and developing countries show that male smoking rates have now peaked and, slowly but surely, are declining. However, this is an extremely slow trend over decades and in the meantime, tobacco is killing nearly 4 million men every year. In general, the higher-educated man is giving up the habit first, so that smoking is becoming a habit of poorer, less educated males.

China deserves special mention because of the enormity of the problem. Consuming more than 30 percent of the world's cigarettes and with almost 70 percent of males still smoking, this huge market is, according to Philip Morris, "the most important feature on the landscape."

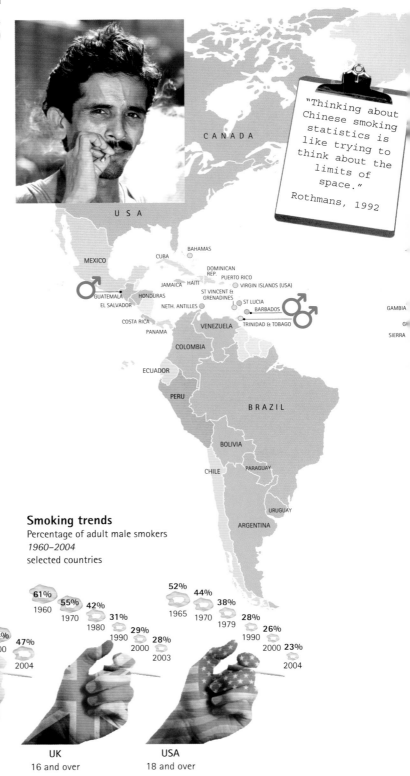

"Thinking about Chinese smoking statistics is like trying to think about the limits of space."
Rothmans, 1992

Smoking trends
Percentage of adult male smokers
1960–2004
selected countries

Japan
20 and over

81% 1960
78% 1970
70% 1980
61% 1990
54% 2000
47% 2004

UK
16 and over

61% 1960
55% 1970
42% 1980
31% 1990
29% 2000
28% 2003

USA
18 and over

52% 1965
44% 1970
38% 1979
28% 1990
26% 2000
23% 2004

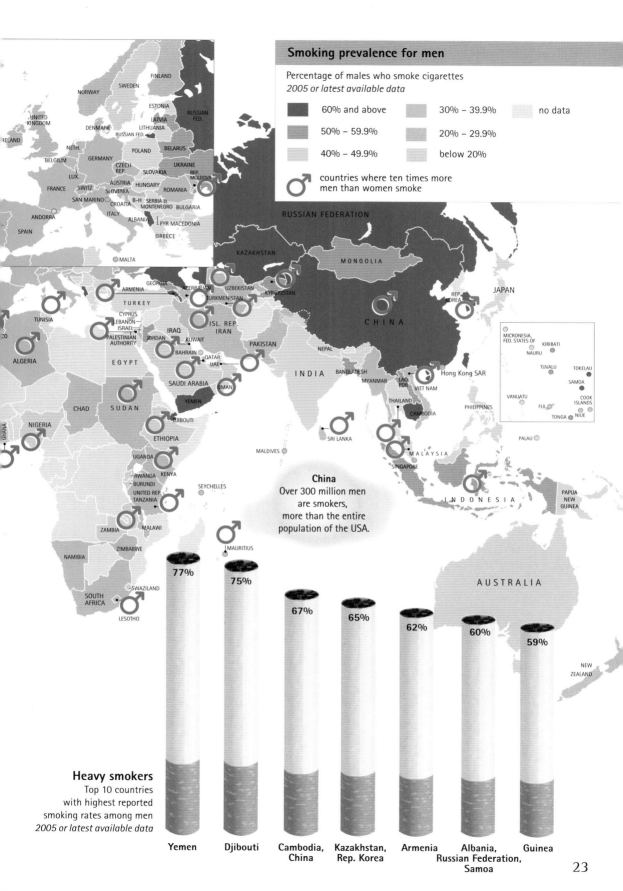

Smoking prevalence for men

Percentage of males who smoke cigarettes
2005 or latest available data

- 60% and above
- 50% – 59.9%
- 40% – 49.9%
- 30% – 39.9%
- 20% – 29.9%
- below 20%
- no data

♂ countries where ten times more men than women smoke

China
Over 300 million men are smokers, more than the entire population of the USA.

Heavy smokers
Top 10 countries with highest reported smoking rates among men
2005 or latest available data

Country	Percentage
Yemen	77%
Djibouti	75%
Cambodia, China	67%
Kazakhstan, Rep. Korea	65%
Armenia	62%
Albania, Russian Federation, Samoa	60%
Guinea	59%

Female smoking

"Women who smoke like men die like men who smoke."
Joseph Califano, US Secretary of Health, Education and Welfare, 1977–79

About 250 million women in the world are daily smokers: 22 percent of women in developed countries, and 9 percent of women in developing countries. In some parts of South Asia, prevalence of oral tobacco use is estimated to be as high as 30 percent in females, compared with 25 percent in males.

Cigarette smoking among women is declining in many developed countries, notably Australia, Canada, the UK and USA, but this trend is not found in all developed countries. In several southern, central and eastern European countries cigarette smoking is either still increasing among women or has not shown any decline.

The tobacco industry promotes cigarettes to women using seductive but false images of vitality, slimness, emancipation, sophistication and sexual allure. In reality, smoking causes reproductive damage, disease and death. Tobacco companies produce a range of brands marketed to women, most notably "women-only" brands: these feminized cigarettes are long, extra-slim, low-tar, light-coloured, or mentholated.

If women start smoking like men, it will be an unmitigated global public health disaster. Preventing an increase in smoking among women in developing countries would have a greater impact than any other health measure.

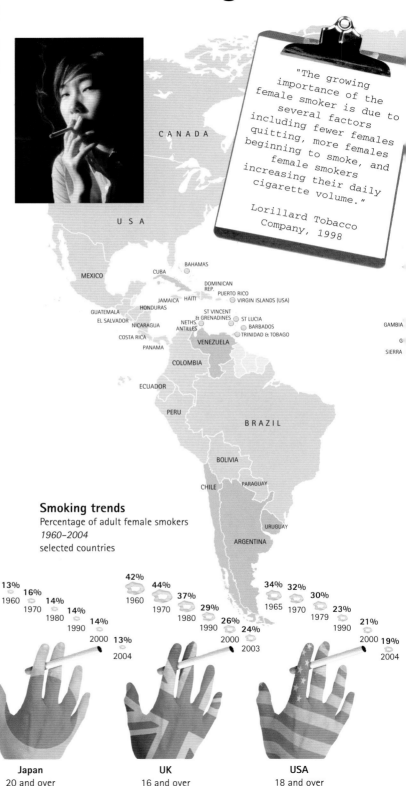

"The growing importance of the female smoker is due to several factors including fewer females quitting, more females beginning to smoke, and female smokers increasing their daily cigarette volume."

Lorillard Tobacco Company, 1998

Smoking trends

Percentage of adult female smokers
1960–2004
selected countries

Japan 20 and over		UK 16 and over		USA 18 and over	
13%	1960	42%	1960	34%	1965
16%	1970	44%	1970	32%	1970
14%	1980	37%	1980	30%	1979
14%	1990	29%	1990	23%	1990
14%	2000	26%	2000	21%	2000
13%	2004	24%	2003	19%	2004

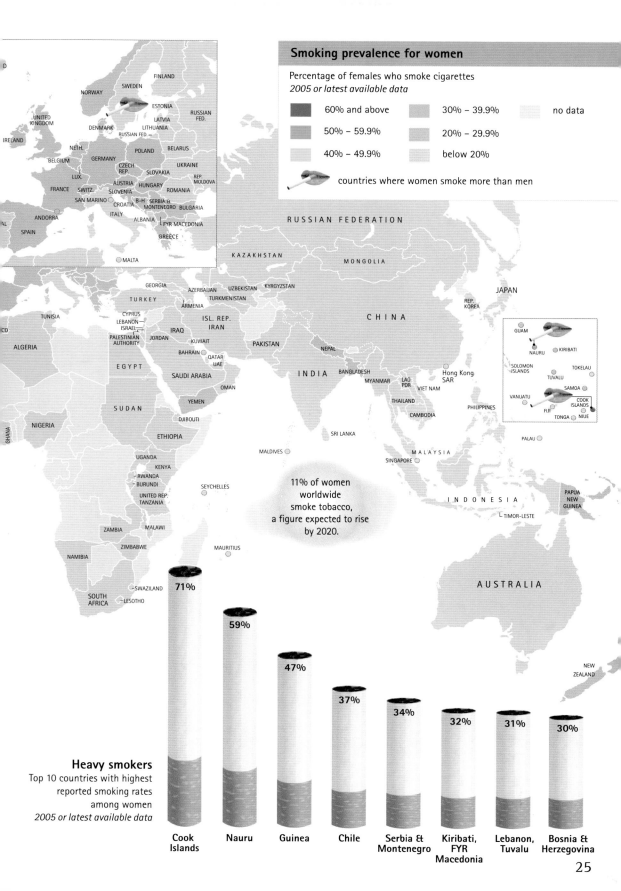

Smoking prevalence for women

Percentage of females who smoke cigarettes
2005 or latest available data

- 60% and above
- 50% – 59.9%
- 40% – 49.9%
- 30% – 39.9%
- 20% – 29.9%
- below 20%
- no data

countries where women smoke more than men

11% of women worldwide smoke tobacco, a figure expected to rise by 2020.

Heavy smokers
Top 10 countries with highest reported smoking rates among women
2005 or latest available data

Country	Percentage
Cook Islands	71%
Nauru	59%
Guinea	47%
Chile	37%
Serbia & Montenegro	34%
Kiribati, FYR Macedonia	32%
Lebanon, Tuvalu	31%
Bosnia & Herzegovina	30%

Health professionals

Whether in the doctor's office, the dentist's chair, or over the pharmacy counter, health professionals have a unique opportunity to counsel individuals on why and how to stop smoking. Even brief advice from a health professional can have a significant impact on smoking cessation rates. However, health professionals who smoke are less likely to help their patients quit smoking and their advice has diminished credibility.

Health-professional smoking prevalence varies widely around the world, reflecting socio-demographic patterns of tobacco use. In early stages of the pandemic, higher status individuals and social trendsetters, such as health professionals, tend to exhibit markedly higher smoking prevalence rates than the general population. In later stages of the pandemic, health professionals – direct observers of the terrible health consequences of long-term smoking – often quit smoking and initiate national tobacco-control movements.

In 2004, a WHO meeting of health professional organizations adopted a code of practice describing 14 ways medical associations could support tobacco control. By quitting their own addiction, becoming proficient at smoking cessation counselling, and by engaging in social and political action against tobacco, health professionals can contribute to reducing tobacco's escalating toll of death and disability.

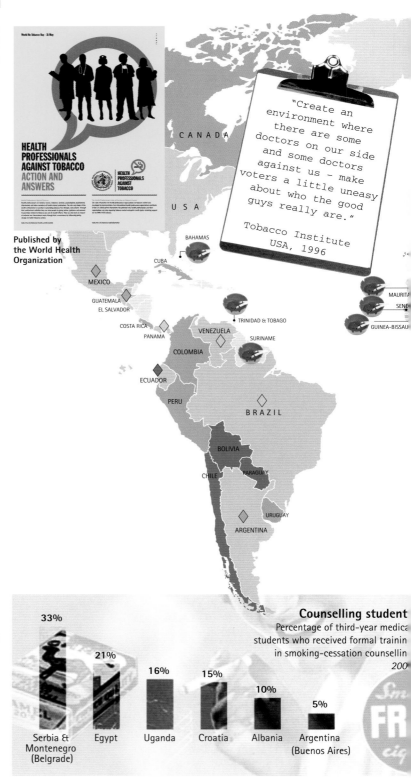

HEALTH PROFESSIONALS AGAINST TOBACCO
ACTION AND ANSWERS

Published by the World Health Organization

"Create an environment where there are some doctors on our side and some doctors against us – make voters a little uneasy about who the good guys really are."
Tobacco Institute USA, 1996

Counselling student
Percentage of third-year medical students who received formal training in smoking-cessation counselling
2003

33% — Serbia & Montenegro (Belgrade)
21% — Egypt
16% — Uganda
15% — Croatia
10% — Albania
5% — Argentina (Buenos Aires)

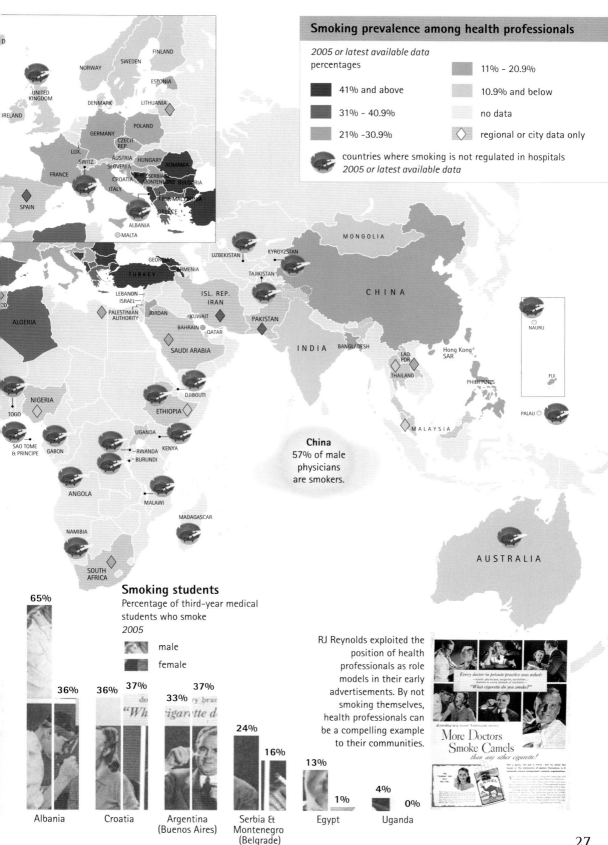

Smoking prevalence among health professionals

2005 or latest available data
percentages

41% and above	11% – 20.9%
31% – 40.9%	10.9% and below
21% –30.9%	no data
	◇ regional or city data only

countries where smoking is not regulated in hospitals
2005 or latest available data

China
57% of male
physicians
are smokers.

Smoking students

Percentage of third-year medical
students who smoke
2005

male

female

65% Albania
36%
36% Croatia
37%
33% Argentina (Buenos Aires)
37%
24% Serbia & Montenegro (Belgrade)
16%
13% Egypt
1%
4% Uganda
0%

RJ Reynolds exploited the
position of health
professionals as role
models in their early
advertisements. By not
smoking themselves,
health professionals can
be a compelling example
to their communities.

27

Boys' tobacco use

The differences in smoking rates between boys and girls are not as large as one would expect. Boys are more likely than girls to smoke but in half the countries covered by the Global Youth Tobacco Survey (GYTS), there was no gender difference. Gender differences in rates of other tobacco use were also minimal; in only 30 percent of countries did boys use other forms of tobacco more than girls.

The overwhelming majority of boys begin using tobacco before they reach adulthood. According to the GYTS, nearly one-quarter of young people who smoke had their first cigarette before the age of ten.

The uptake of smoking among boys increases with tobacco industry promotion, easy access to tobacco products, low prices, peer pressure, their peers, parents and siblings using tobacco and approving of smoking, and the misperception that smoking enhances social popularity.

While the most serious health effects of tobacco consumption normally occur after decades of smoking, tobacco also causes immediate health effects for young smokers. Perhaps more importantly, teenage smokers risk addiction while in adolescence. Smokers who become addicted to tobacco in their youth face the greatest risk of eventually contracting diseases caused by smoking, such as cancer, emphysema and heart disease.

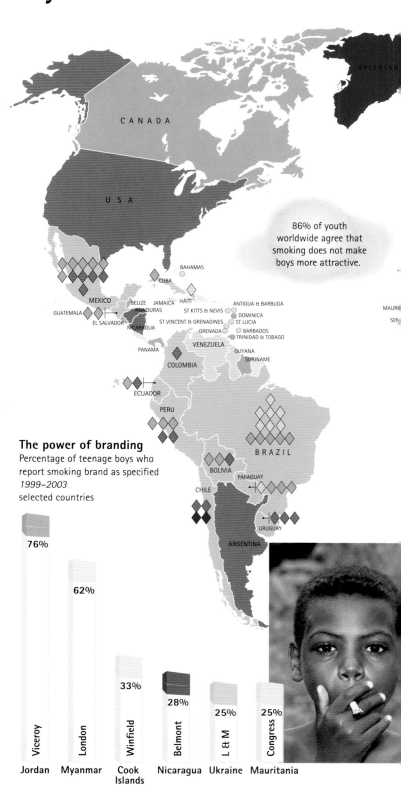

86% of youth worldwide agree that smoking does not make boys more attractive.

The power of branding
Percentage of teenage boys who report smoking brand as specified
1999–2003
selected countries

Brand	%
Viceroy — Jordan	76%
London — Myanmar	62%
Winfield — Cook Islands	33%
Belmont — Nicaragua	28%
L & M — Ukraine	25%
Congress — Mauritania	25%

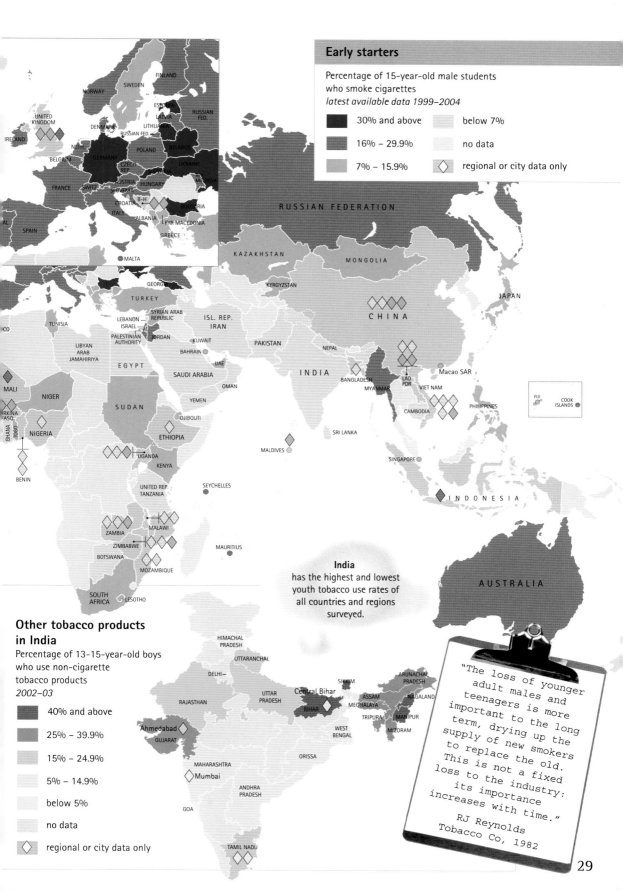

Percentage of 15-year-old male students
who smoke cigarettes
latest available data 1999–2004

- 30% and above
- 16% – 29.9%
- 7% – 15.9%
- below 7%
- no data
- ◇ regional or city data only

RUSSIAN FEDERATION

India
has the highest and lowest
youth tobacco use rates of
all countries and regions
surveyed.

Other tobacco products in India

Percentage of 13–15-year-old boys
who use non-cigarette
tobacco products
2002–03

- 40% and above
- 25% – 39.9%
- 15% – 24.9%
- 5% – 14.9%
- below 5%
- no data
- ◇ regional or city data only

"The loss of younger
adult males and
teenagers is more
important to the long
term, drying up the
supply of new smokers
to replace the old.
This is not a fixed
loss to the industry:
its importance
increases with time."
RJ Reynolds
Tobacco Co, 1982

29

Girls' tobacco use

The differences in smoking rates between girls and boys are not as large as one would expect. In half of countries surveyed in the Global Youth Tobacco Survey (GYTS), there were no gender differences in cigarette smoking. Similarly, in 70 percent of countries surveyed, there were no differences in other tobacco use. Worldwide, tobacco use among girls is increasing, and in parts of Europe and South America, girls are smoking more than boys. As with boys, the overwhelming majority of female smokers use tobacco before they reach adulthood.

The factors that increase the risk of girls smoking are broadly similar to those of boys: tobacco industry promotion, easy access to tobacco products, low prices, peer pressure, their peers, parents and siblings using tobacco and approving of smoking, and the misperception that smoking enhances social popularity.

In addition, young girls smoke to stay thin, although cigarette smoking is not associated with a lower BMI (body mass index) in younger women. Smoking prevention and cessation programmes designed for girls may benefit from the inclusion of content related to body image.

Reasons why more young women smoke

- global trends in women's emancipation
- greater concern with weight, looks and style
- marketing campaigns targeting women
- positive images of smoking in movies, magazines and youth culture
- changing economic conditions for some women
- a more drug-positive culture in some countries

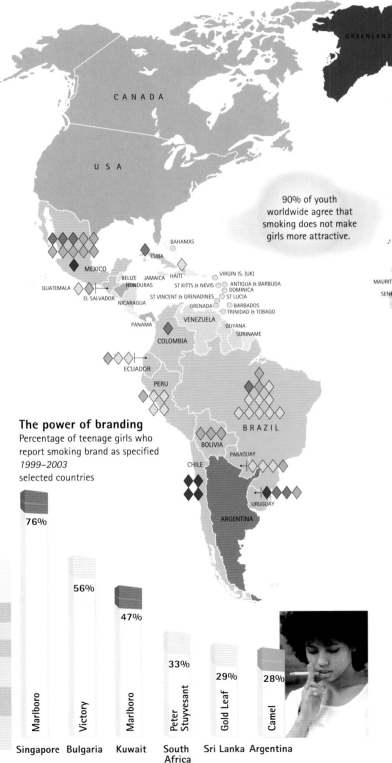

90% of youth worldwide agree that smoking does not make girls more attractive.

The power of branding
Percentage of teenage girls who report smoking brand as specified
1999–2003
selected countries

76%	56%	47%	33%	29%	28%
Marlboro	Victory	Marlboro	Peter Stuyvesant	Gold Leaf	Camel
Singapore	Bulgaria	Kuwait	South Africa	Sri Lanka	Argentina

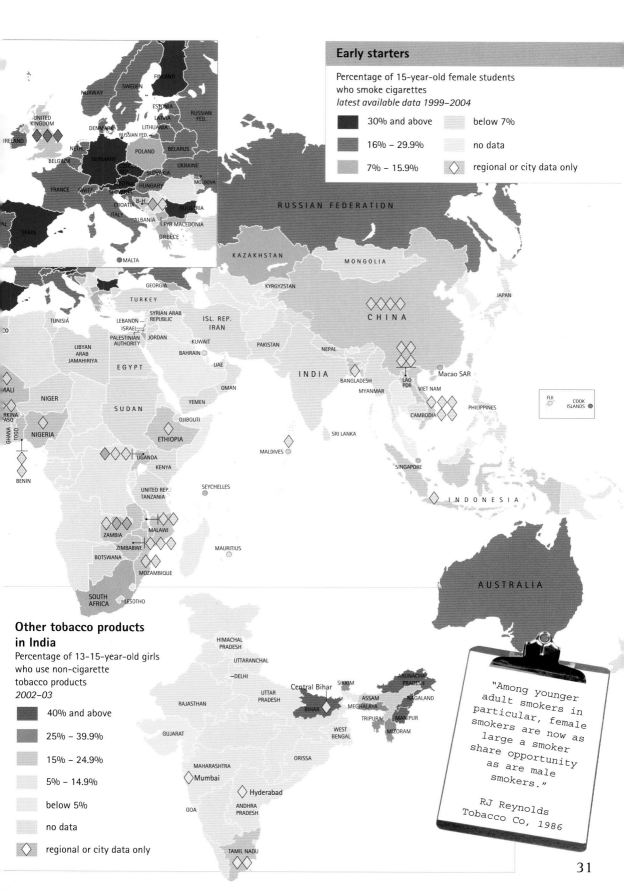

Early starters

Percentage of 15-year-old female students who smoke cigarettes
latest available data 1999–2004

- 30% and above
- 16% – 29.9%
- 7% – 15.9%
- below 7%
- no data
- ◇ regional or city data only

Other tobacco products in India

Percentage of 13-15-year-old girls who use non-cigarette tobacco products
2002–03

- 40% and above
- 25% – 39.9%
- 15% – 24.9%
- 5% – 14.9%
- below 5%
- no data
- ◇ regional or city data only

"Among younger adult smokers in particular, female smokers are now as large a smoker share opportunity as are male smokers."

RJ Reynolds Tobacco Co, 1986

Cigarette consumption

> "A cigarette is the perfect type of a perfect pleasure. It is exquisite, and leaves one unsatisfied. What more could one want?"
> Oscar Wilde, *The Picture of Dorian Gray*, 1890

Global cigarette consumption has been rising steadily since James Bonsack invented the first cigarette-rolling machine in 1881. By the 1960s, the incontrovertible health consequences of smoking had become apparent and, in some countries, consumption began levelling off and even decreasing. Worldwide, however, more people are smoking, and each smoker is consuming a greater number of cigarettes. Cigarettes account for the largest share of manufactured tobacco products (96 percent of total value sales) but widespread consumption of chewing tobacco and bidis is also escalating, especially in South Asia.

The total number of smokers is increasing mainly due to expansion of the world's population; by 2030, there will be at least another 2 billion people. Unless smoking prevalence rates decline dramatically, the absolute number of smokers will increase. The expected continuing decrease in male smoking prevalence also may be offset, in part, by a potentially dangerous increase in female smoking rates, especially in developing countries.

Tobacco companies are producing 5.6 trillion cigarettes per year — nearly 900 cigarettes per year for every man, woman, and child on the planet. The escalating consumption of these tobacco products has created an unprecedented global public health emergency, a pandemic of epic proportions.

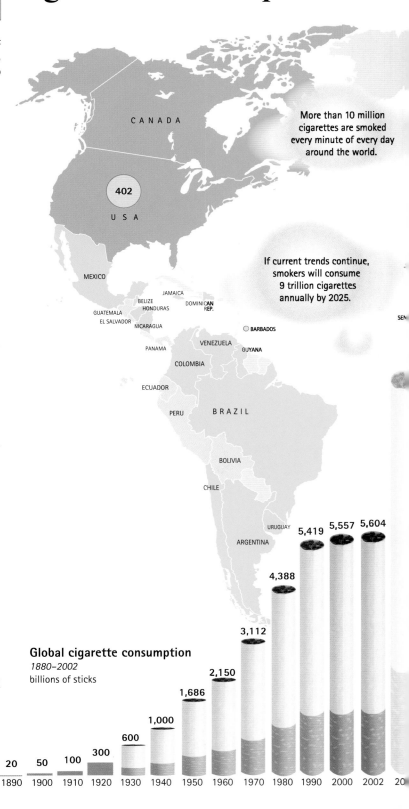

More than 10 million cigarettes are smoked every minute of every day around the world.

If current trends continue, smokers will consume 9 trillion cigarettes annually by 2025.

Global cigarette consumption
1880–2002
billions of sticks

	1880	1890	1900	1910	1920	1930	1940	1950	1960	1970	1980	1990	2000	2002
	10	20	50	100	300	600	1,000	1,686	2,150	3,112	4,388	5,419	5,557	5,604

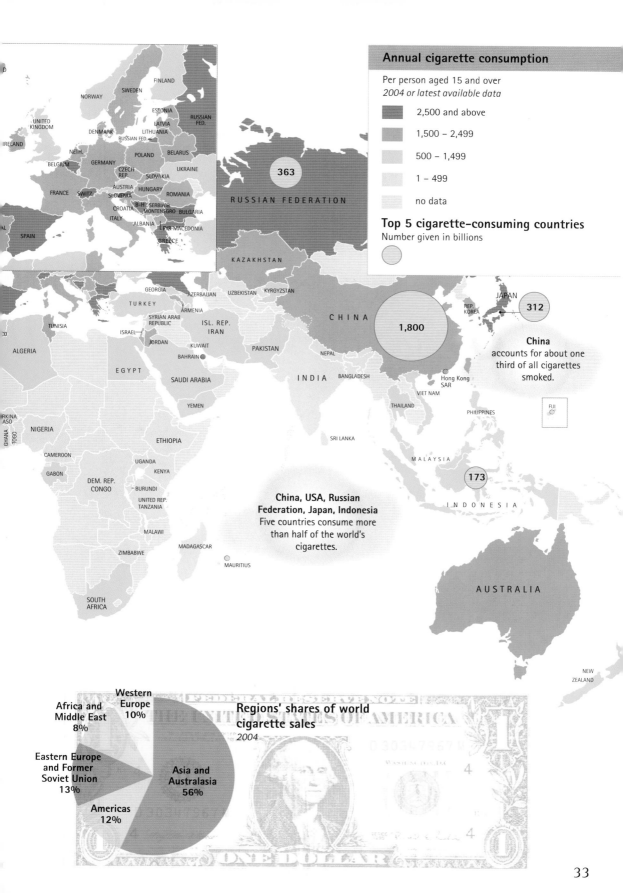

Annual cigarette consumption

Per person aged 15 and over
2004 or latest available data

2,500 and above

1,500 – 2,499

500 – 1,499

1 – 499

no data

Top 5 cigarette-consuming countries

Number given in billions

RUSSIAN FEDERATION 363

CHINA 1,800

JAPAN 312

INDONESIA 173

China accounts for about one third of all cigarettes smoked.

China, USA, Russian Federation, Japan, Indonesia
Five countries consume more than half of the world's cigarettes.

Regions' shares of world cigarette sales
2004

- Western Europe 10%
- Africa and Middle East 8%
- Eastern Europe and Former Soviet Union 13%
- Americas 12%
- Asia and Australasia 56%

Health risks

All forms of tobacco are addictive and lethal. Conclusive scientific evidence confirms that smokers face significantly increased risks of death from numerous cancers (particularly lung cancer), heart disease, stroke, emphysema and many other fatal and non-fatal diseases. Cigar, pipe, waterpipe and bidi smokers suffer the same types of health consequences as cigarette smokers. Those who chew tobacco face greatly elevated risks for cancers of the oral cavity, especially of the lip, tongue, palate and pharynx.

Women and children suffer additional health risks from smoking. Smoking during pregnancy is dangerous to the mother as well as to the foetus, and may result in developmental problems that haunt children throughout their lives. Exposure to second-hand smoke during childhood compounds the adverse effects of foetal exposure.

Cigarettes low in tar or nicotine do not reduce smoking hazards. However, quitting greatly reduces health risks and produces immediate and long-term health benefits. From a public health perspective, tobacco has virtually no positive attributes. Nicotine is used as an insecticide and researchers continue to seek other uses for the tobacco plant, such as genetic engineering or growing biomass.

Health risks due to smoking in pregnancy

Mother:
Spontaneous abortion / miscarriage
Ectopic pregnancy
Abruptio placentae
Placenta praevia
Premature rupture of the membranes
Premature birth

Foetus, infants, children:
Smaller infant (for gestational age)
Stillborn infant
Birth defects, e.g. oral clefts and limb reduction
Sudden Infant Death Syndrome (SIDS)
Reduced lung function
Long-term physical and mental effects
Lower respiratory tract infections

Deadly chemicals
Tobacco smoke contains over 4,000 chemicals, 60 of which are known or suspected carcinogens and some of which have marked irritant properties.

Tobacco smoke includes	as found in
Acetone	paint stripper
Arsenic	ant poison
Butane	lighter fuel
Cadmium	car batteries
Carbon monoxide	car exhaust fumes
DDT	insecticide
Formaldehyde	embalming fluid
Hydrogen cyanide	capital punishment by gas
Methanol	rocket fuel
Nicotine	cockroach poison
Phenol	toilet bowl disinfectant
Propylene glycol	antifreeze
Toluene	industrial solvent
Vinyl chloride	plastics

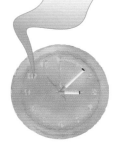

Time ticks away
Every cigarette takes 7 minutes off a smoker's life.

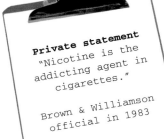

Private statement
"Nicotine is the addicting agent in cigarettes."

Brown & Williamson official in 1983

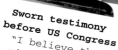

Sworn testimony before US Congress
"I believe that nicotine is not addictive."

CEOs of the seven leading tobacco companies in 1994

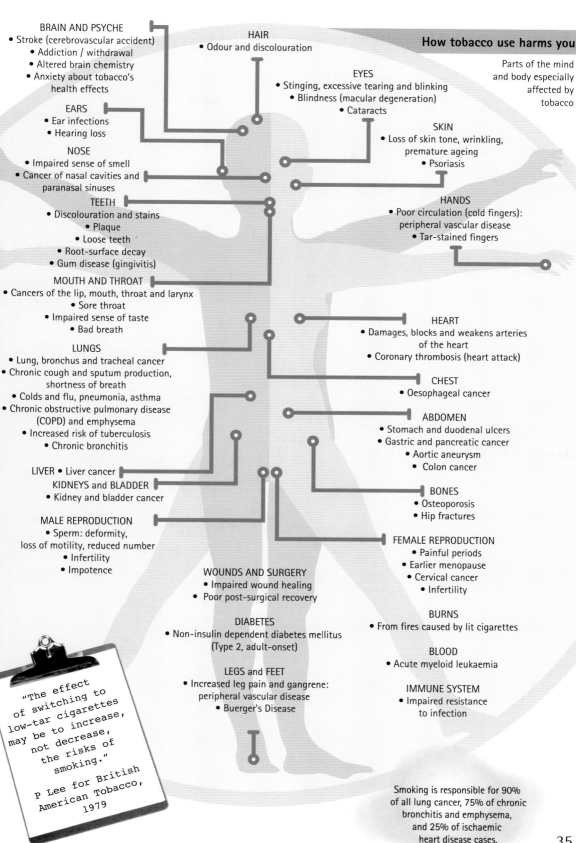

BRAIN AND PSYCHE
- Stroke (cerebrovascular accident)
  - Addiction / withdrawal
  - Altered brain chemistry
  - Anxiety about tobacco's
    health effects

HAIR
- Odour and discolouration

How tobacco use harms you

Parts of the mind
and body especially
affected by
tobacco

EYES
- Stinging, excessive tearing and blinking
  - Blindness (macular degeneration)
    - Cataracts

EARS
- Ear infections
- Hearing loss

SKIN
- Loss of skin tone, wrinkling,
  premature ageing
  - Psoriasis

NOSE
- Impaired sense of smell
- Cancer of nasal cavities and
  paranasal sinuses

HANDS
- Poor circulation (cold fingers):
  peripheral vascular disease
  - Tar-stained fingers

TEETH
- Discolouration and stains
  - Plaque
  - Loose teeth
  - Root-surface decay
  - Gum disease (gingivitis)

MOUTH AND THROAT
- Cancers of the lip, mouth, throat and larynx
  - Sore throat
  - Impaired sense of taste
  - Bad breath

HEART
- Damages, blocks and weakens arteries
  of the heart
  - Coronary thrombosis (heart attack)

LUNGS
- Lung, bronchus and tracheal cancer
- Chronic cough and sputum production,
  shortness of breath
  - Colds and flu, pneumonia, asthma
- Chronic obstructive pulmonary disease
  (COPD) and emphysema
  - Increased risk of tuberculosis
    - Chronic bronchitis

CHEST
- Oesophageal cancer

ABDOMEN
- Stomach and duodenal ulcers
- Gastric and pancreatic cancer
  - Aortic aneurysm
    - Colon cancer

LIVER • Liver cancer
KIDNEYS and BLADDER
- Kidney and bladder cancer

BONES
- Osteoporosis
- Hip fractures

MALE REPRODUCTION
- Sperm: deformity,
  loss of motility, reduced number
  - Infertility
  - Impotence

FEMALE REPRODUCTION
- Painful periods
- Earlier menopause
- Cervical cancer
- Infertility

WOUNDS AND SURGERY
- Impaired wound healing
- Poor post-surgical recovery

BURNS
- From fires caused by lit cigarettes

DIABETES
- Non-insulin dependent diabetes mellitus
  (Type 2, adult-onset)

BLOOD
- Acute myeloid leukaemia

LEGS and FEET
- Increased leg pain and gangrene:
  peripheral vascular disease
  - Buerger's Disease

IMMUNE SYSTEM
- Impaired resistance
  to infection

"The effect
of switching to
low-tar cigarettes
may be to increase,
not decrease,
the risks of
smoking."

P Lee for British
American Tobacco,
1979

Smoking is responsible for 90%
of all lung cancer, 75% of chronic
bronchitis and emphysema,
and 25% of ischaemic
heart disease cases.

Passive smoking

9

> "An hour a day in a room with a smoker is nearly a hundred times more likely to cause lung cancer in a non-smoker than twenty years spent in a building containing asbestos."
> Sir Richard Doll, 1985

Passive smoking is also known as exposure to second-hand smoke (SHS) or environmental tobacco smoke (ETS). A passive smoker breathes "sidestream" smoke from the burning tip of the cigarette and "mainstream" smoke that has been exhaled by the smoker. Sidestream smoke is the major component of SHS and is more toxic per unit of tobacco than mainstream smoke.

Passive smoking causes a variety of adverse health effects in non-smokers. Non-smokers exposed to second-hand smoke have an increased lung cancer risk of between 20 percent and 30 percent, and a 25 percent increased risk of heart disease. In addition to harming the mother, passive smoking during pregnancy is linked to health problems in the foetus and infant.

Growing evidence about the health risks of passive smoking has prompted many countries to ban smoking in public areas. While such bans are important and necessary steps to protect non-smokers from second-hand smoke, they are not sufficient to protect young people from the harm caused by exposure to tobacco smoke. Almost half of the world's children are exposed to tobacco smoke, the majority of them in the home. To secure every child's right to grow up in an environment free of tobacco smoke, adult smoking rates must be reduced, especially among parents.

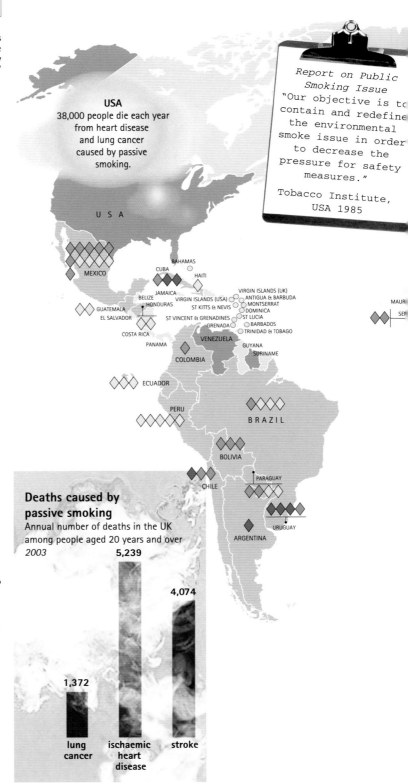

USA
38,000 people die each year from heart disease and lung cancer caused by passive smoking.

> Report on Public Smoking Issue
> "Our objective is to contain and redefine the environmental smoke issue in order to decrease the pressure for safety measures."
> Tobacco Institute, USA 1985

Deaths caused by passive smoking
Annual number of deaths in the UK among people aged 20 years and over
2003

5,239	
4,074	
1,372	

lung cancer | ischaemic heart disease | stroke

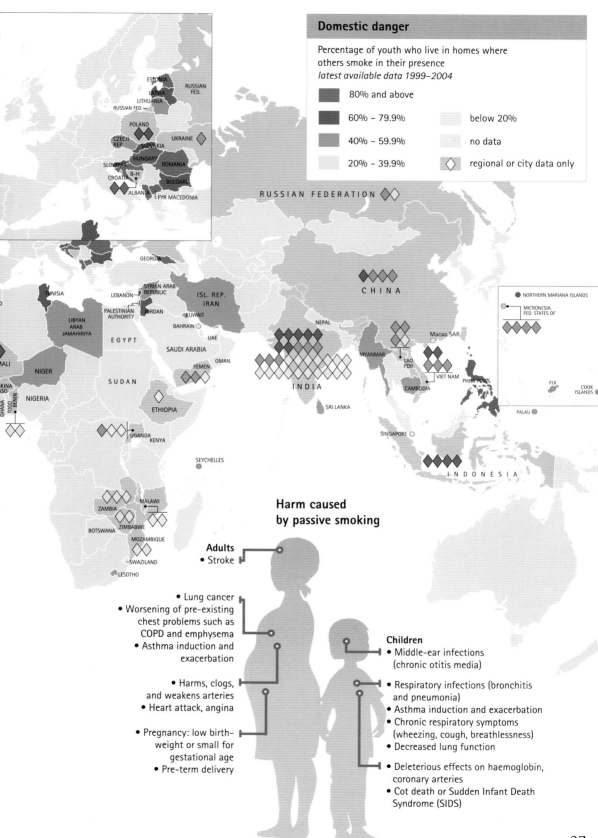

Domestic danger

Percentage of youth who live in homes where others smoke in their presence
latest available data 1999–2004

- 80% and above
- 60% – 79.9%
- 40% – 59.9%
- 20% – 39.9%
- below 20%
- no data
- regional or city data only

Harm caused by passive smoking

Adults
- Stroke
- Lung cancer
- Worsening of pre-existing chest problems such as COPD and emphysema
- Asthma induction and exacerbation
- Harms, clogs, and weakens arteries
- Heart attack, angina
- Pregnancy: low birth-weight or small for gestational age
- Pre-term delivery

Children
- Middle-ear infections (chronic otitis media)
- Respiratory infections (bronchitis and pneumonia)
- Asthma induction and exacerbation
- Chronic respiratory symptoms (wheezing, cough, breathlessness)
- Decreased lung function
- Deleterious effects on haemoglobin, coronary arteries
- Cot death or Sudden Infant Death Syndrome (SIDS)

Tobacco use, in any form, is deadly. Smoking kills half of all lifetime users and half of those deaths occur between the ages of 30 and 69. If current smoking patterns continue, tobacco will kill about 10 million people every year by 2020 and 70 percent of these deaths will occur in developing nations.

Smoking accounts for 12 percent of global adult mortality with more men dying from smoking in developing countries than in industrialized countries. Currently, more men than women die from smoking, but smoking rates are increasing among women in many developing countries.

Tobacco also causes deaths among non-smokers. Maternal smoking during pregnancy is responsible for many foetal deaths and is also a major cause of Sudden Infant Death Syndrome. Exposure to secondhand smoke in the home, workplace, and public areas also kills tens of thousands of non-smokers every year. Infants, children, pregnant women and foetuses are at particularly high risk from secondhand smoke.

One hundred million people died from tobacco use in the 20th century. Unless effective measures are implemented to prevent young people from smoking and to help current users quit, tobacco will kill 1 billion people in the 21st century.

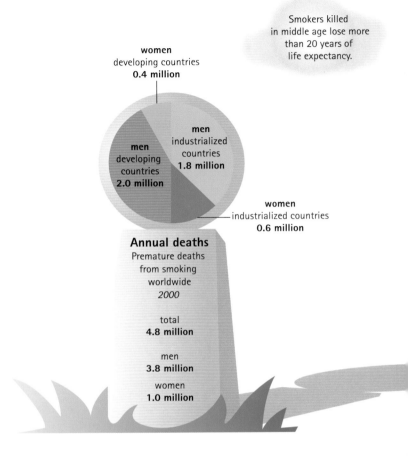

Smokers killed in middle age lose more than 20 years of life expectancy.

women developing countries
0.4 million

men industrialized countries
1.8 million

men developing countries
2.0 million

women industrialized countries
0.6 million

Annual deaths
Premature deaths from smoking worldwide
2000

total
4.8 million

men
3.8 million

women
1.0 million

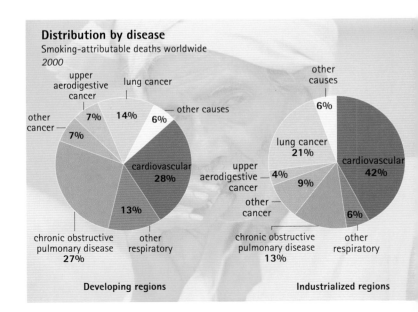

Distribution by disease
Smoking-attributable deaths worldwide
2000

upper aerodigestive cancer
7%

lung cancer
14%

other causes
6%

other cancer
7%

cardiovascular
28%

chronic obstructive pulmonary disease
27%

other respiratory
13%

Developing regions

other causes
6%

lung cancer
21%

cardiovascular
42%

upper aerodigestive cancer
4%

9%

other cancer

chronic obstructive pulmonary disease
13%

other respiratory
6%

Industrialized regions

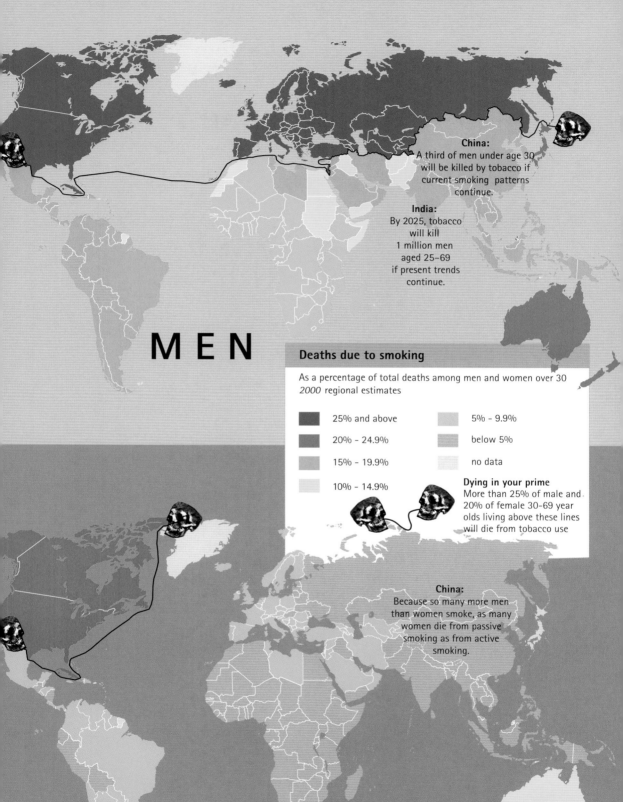

MEN

China:
A third of men under age 30 will be killed by tobacco if current smoking patterns continue.

India:
By 2025, tobacco will kill 1 million men aged 25–69 if present trends continue.

Deaths due to smoking

As a percentage of total deaths among men and women over 30
2000 regional estimates

- 25% and above
- 20% – 24.9%
- 15% – 19.9%
- 10% – 14.9%
- 5% – 9.9%
- below 5%
- no data

Dying in your prime
More than 25% of male and 20% of female 30-69 year olds living above these lines will die from tobacco use

China:
Because so many more men than women smoke, as many women die from passive smoking as from active smoking.

WOMEN

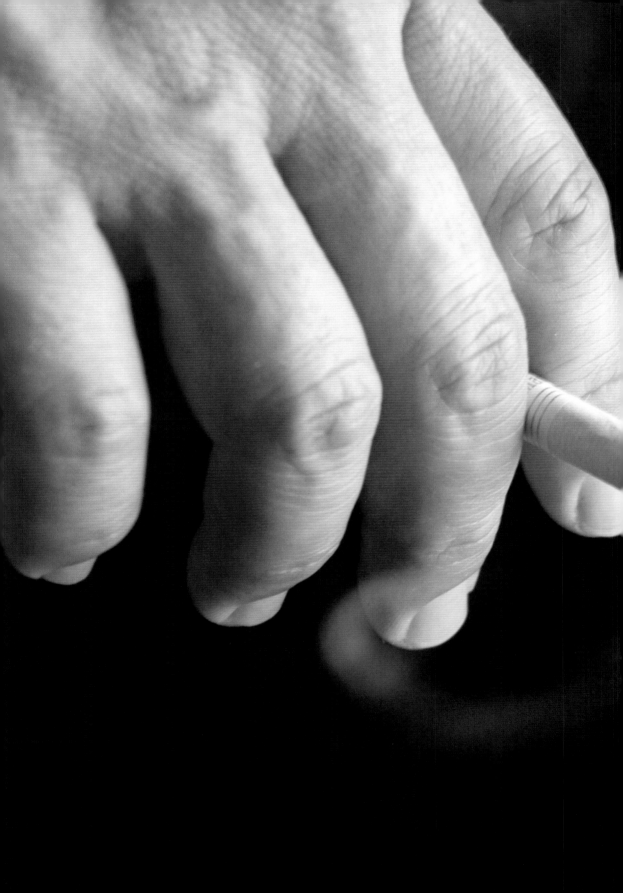

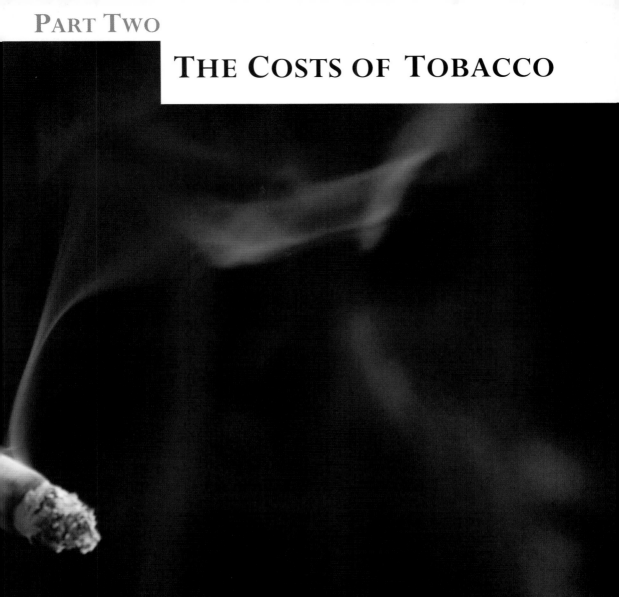

PART TWO

THE COSTS OF TOBACCO

"Tobacco control, rather than being a luxury that only
rich nations can afford, is now a necessity that all
countries must address."

Conclusion of the WHO's report *Tobacco and Poverty: A Vicious Cycle*, 2004

Costs to the economy

Tobacco companies frequently attempt to persuade governmental authorities and the public that smoking has economic benefits. They claim that tobacco control measures will reduce tax revenues, increase unemployment, and even that non-smokers who live longer will create great hardships for national economies. Yet the industry studiously neglects to mention that tobacco imposes enormous economic costs on every country.

Tobacco's burden on governments, employers and the environment are largely hidden taxes, including hugely increased healthcare costs, loss of foreign exchange for imported cigarettes, diversion of agricultural land that could grow food, the costs of fires and damage to buildings caused by careless smokers, the resulting increase in insurance premiums, employee absenteeism, decreased worker productivity, and widespread environmental costs due to large-scale deforestation, pesticide and fertilizer pollution, and the millions of discarded butts and cigarette packaging that litter streets and waterways.

As tobacco is an important cash crop in some countries, Article 17 of the World Health Organization's Framework Convention on Tobacco Control urges countries to promote economically viable alternatives for those involved in tobacco production. Economic incentives can encourage tobacco farmers and

workers involved in cigarette manufacturing and distribution to shift towards more productive types of employment, improving overall public welfare without sacrificing livelihoods or creating undue hardship. With the numbers of smokers set to rise, this process will occur over many decades.

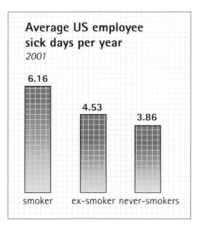

US$184.54 billion

CANADA

US$12.89 billion

U S A

US$97 million

PUERTO RICO

US$284 million

VENEZUELA

Every year children start 1,000,000 fires using cigarette lighters.

Average US employee sick days per year
2001

6.16

4.53

3.86

smoker ex-smoker never-smokers

"...reflecting 5.23 years of life lost for the average smoker – indirect positive effects [are that] public finance benefits from smoking indirectly, via savings on the healthcare costs – in pensions – and public housing costs savings."

Report on the Czech Republic, commissioned by Philip Morris, 2001

UK
In 2005,
the average damage
caused by a house fire
cost £25,300.

Economic costs

Economic costs attributable to tobacco use *2005 or latest available data*

○ direct healthcare costs

◎ total costs
*direct healthcare costs plus indirect economic burden, including
productivity loss, absenteeism, and other socio-economic costs*

▪ no data

US$1.62
billion

US$2.30
billion
NORWAY

US$240
million
FINLAND

US$828
million
DENMARK

UNITED
KINGDOM

US$2.93
billion
NETHERLANDS

GERMANY

US$24.38
billion

FRANCE

US$9.58
billion
SWITZERLAND

US$4.29
billion
C H I N A

US$3.33
billion
REP.
KOREA

US$16.44
billion

US$63.16
million
I N D I A

BANGLADESH

Hong Kong SAR

US$33.80
million

US$424
million

More than 1.6 million
cigarette butts
were collected in and along
the world's coasts and
waterways in 2003.

US$103
million
SOUTH
AFRICA

Trash collected
along the world's coasts
91 countries *2003*

cigarette litter
(including packaging
and filters)
34%

other
66%

USA
Between 1997-2001,
tobacco smoking resulted
in $92 billion of annual
productivity losses.

AUSTRALIA

US$14.19
billion

NEW
ZEALAND

USA
Smoking accounted
for over 6%
of total healthcare expenses
in 1999.

US$17.03
billion

Cost of fires caused by smoking
worldwide
2000

- percentage of all fire deaths: 10%
- total killed by fires caused by
  smoking: 300,000
- total cost of fires caused by smoking:
  US$27 billion

Cost of fires caused by smoking
in the USA
2002

- 14,450 residential fires caused by
  smoking
- 520 deaths
- 1,330 injuries
- $371 million in residential property
  damage

43

Costs to the smoker

> "Smoking makes the poor poorer, it takes away not just health but wealth."
> Dr Bill O'Neill, Secretary of the British Medical Association Scotland, 2004

Smokers waste vast amounts of money on their tobacco addiction that could otherwise be invested in productive economic activity or used to obtain food, clothes and education. In poverty-stricken households where a large proportion of the household income is spent on food, tobacco addiction can lead to malnutrition for the smoker's family.

Smokers also may suffer significant loss of income due to illness, and ill health can trigger a slide into extreme poverty. Tobacco kills one quarter of all smokers during their most productive years of employment, depriving their families of vital income. Family members must expend valuable time and scarce resources caring for their sick and dying smoking relatives. In many developing countries, a visit to the hospital can consume days of travel and a family's life savings.

Smokers must shoulder higher health insurance premiums and many other miscellaneous costs, such as increased wear and tear on their home, as well as increased fire risk.

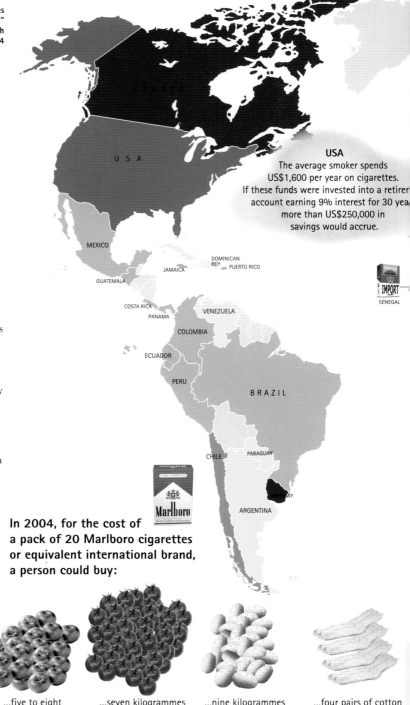

USA
The average smoker spends US$1,600 per year on cigarettes. If these funds were invested into a retirer account earning 9% interest for 30 yea more than US$250,000 in savings would accrue.

In 2004, for the cost of a pack of 20 Marlboro cigarettes or equivalent international brand, a person could buy:

...two and a half small fish in **Sri Lanka**...

...ten litres of milk in **Algeria**...

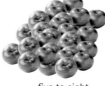

...five to eight kilogrammes of apples in **Armenia**...

...seven kilogrammes of tomatoes in **Jordan**...

...nine kilogrammes of potatoes in **Armenia** and **Uruguay**...

...four pairs of cotton socks in **Lao People's Democratic Republic.**

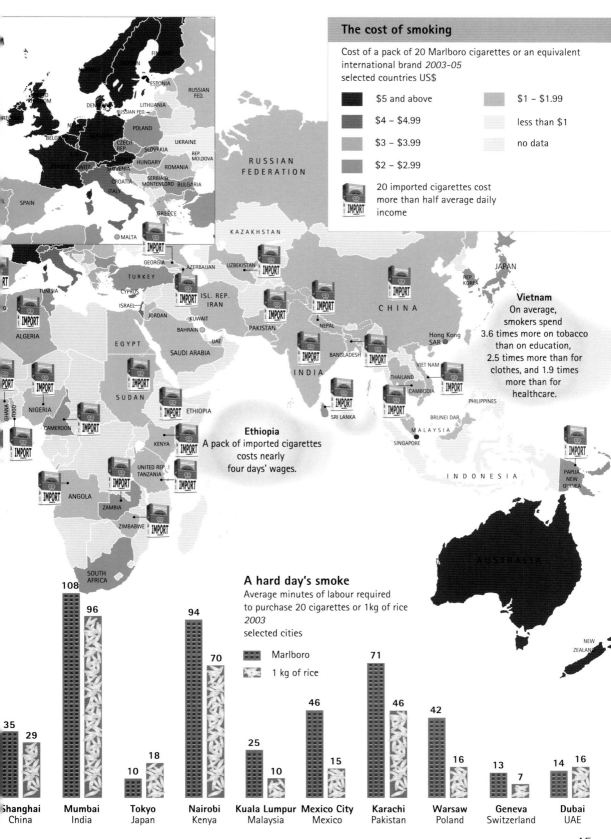

The cost of smoking

Cost of a pack of 20 Marlboro cigarettes or an equivalent international brand *2003-05*
selected countries US$

- $5 and above
- $4 – $4.99
- $3 – $3.99
- $2 – $2.99
- $1 – $1.99
- less than $1
- no data

IMPORT 20 imported cigarettes cost more than half average daily income

Vietnam
On average, smokers spend 3.6 times more on tobacco than on education, 2.5 times more than for clothes, and 1.9 times more than for healthcare.

Ethiopia
A pack of imported cigarettes costs nearly four days' wages.

A hard day's smoke
Average minutes of labour required to purchase 20 cigarettes or 1kg of rice *2003*
selected cities

- Marlboro
- 1 kg of rice

City	Marlboro	1 kg of rice
Shanghai, China	35	29
Mumbai, India	108	96
Tokyo, Japan	10	18
Nairobi, Kenya	94	70
Kuala Lumpur, Malaysia	25	10
Mexico City, Mexico	46	15
Karachi, Pakistan	71	46
Warsaw, Poland	42	16
Geneva, Switzerland	13	7
Dubai, UAE	14	16

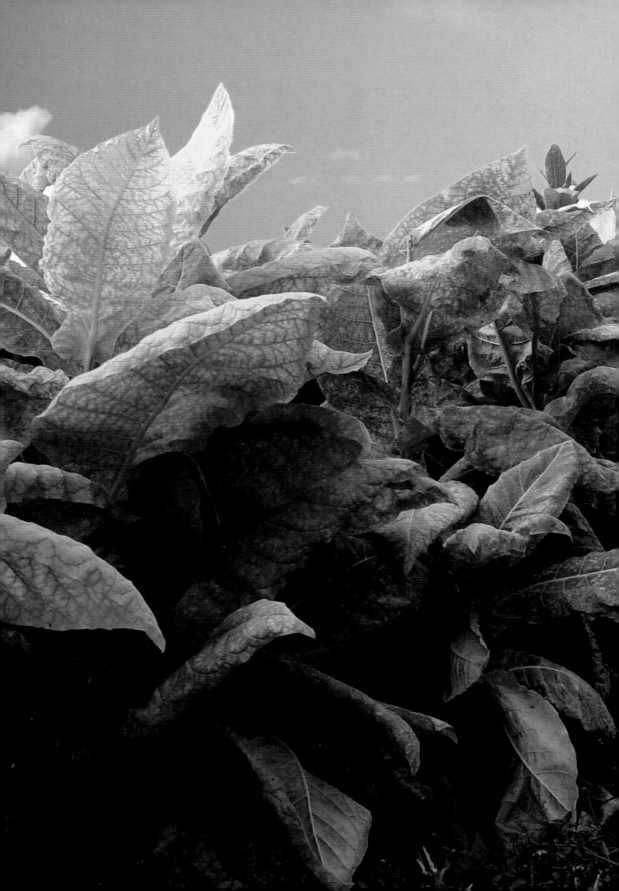

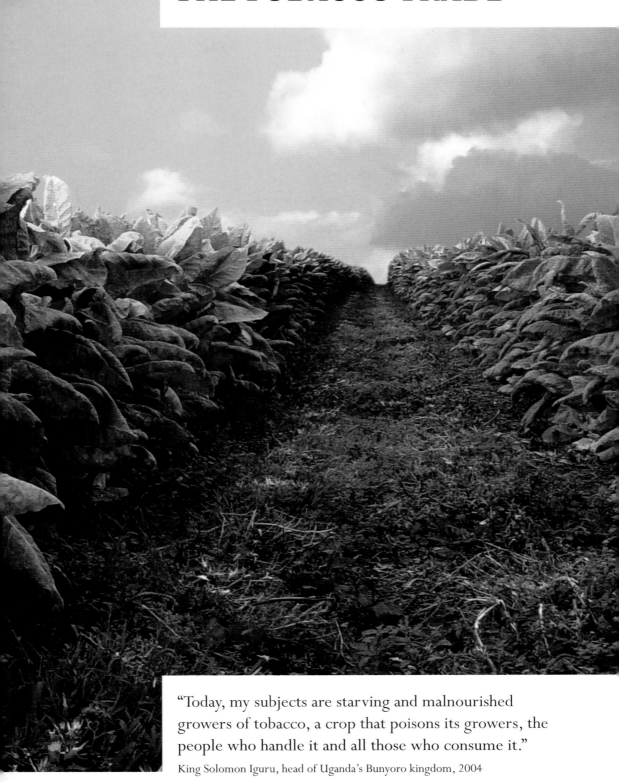

THE TOBACCO TRADE

"Today, my subjects are starving and malnourished growers of tobacco, a crop that poisons its growers, the people who handle it and all those who consume it."

King Solomon Iguru, head of Uganda's Bunyoro kingdom, 2004

13 | Growing tobacco

Tobacco is grown in over 120 countries on more than 4 million hectares of the world's agricultural land.

Globally, tobacco production has almost doubled since the 1960s, totalling nearly 6.5 million metric tonnes in 2004. In developing countries, increasing demand and favourable policies have resulted in a threefold increase in production, while production has declined by more than 50 percent in developed countries. If this trend continues as projected to 2010, more than 85 percent of the world's tobacco will be grown in developing countries.

Tobacco agriculture causes widespread environmental and public health problems. Pesticide and fertilizer runoff from fields and massive deforestation associated with tobacco curing damage the environment. Workers suffer pesticide poisoning, Green Tobacco Sickness (an occupational hazard unique to tobacco), and lung damage from exposure to tobacco and field dust.

Although tobacco farming is very profitable for multinational corporations, many small farmers are caught in a debt trap perpetuated by the tobacco companies.

The WHO's Framework Convention on Tobacco Control calls for financial and technical assistance to tobacco growers in countries, such as Zimbabwe and Malawi, heavily dependent on tobacco agriculture. Shifting to economically viable and environmentally sound agricultural alternatives promises a healthier future for tobacco-producing nations.

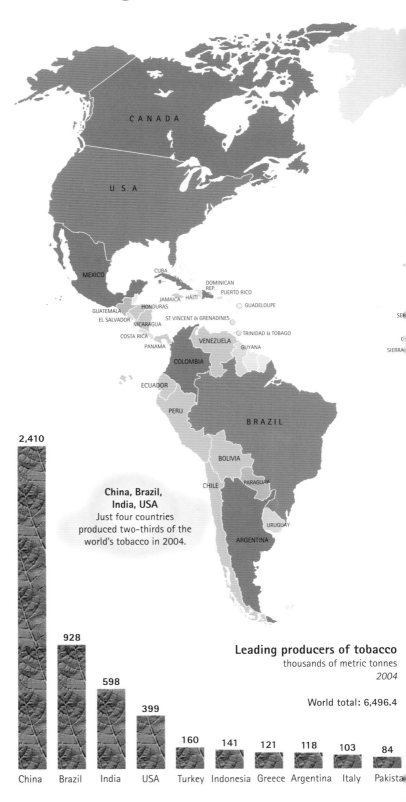

China, Brazil, India, USA
Just four countries produced two-thirds of the world's tobacco in 2004.

Leading producers of tobacco
thousands of metric tonnes
2004

World total: 6,496.4

China	Brazil	India	USA	Turkey	Indonesia	Greece	Argentina	Italy	Pakistan
2,410	928	598	399	160	141	121	118	103	84

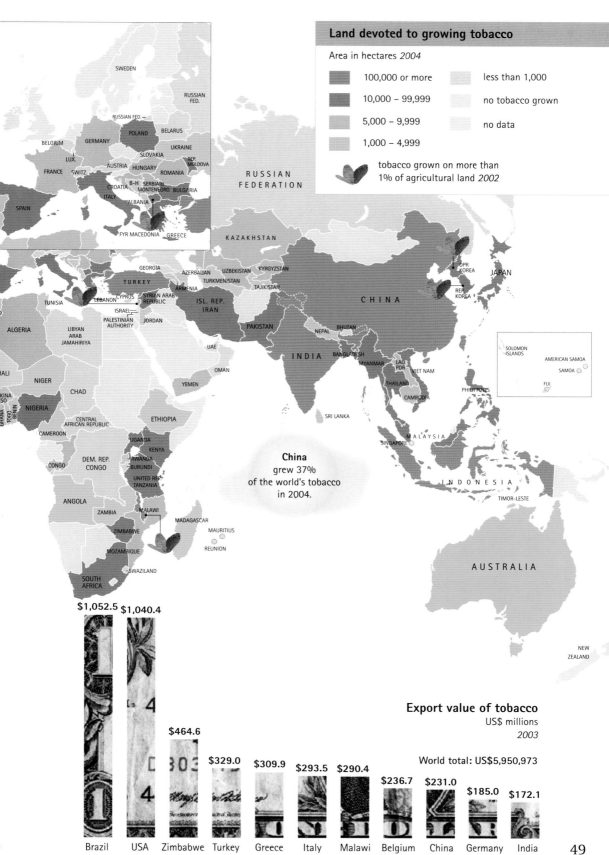

Land devoted to growing tobacco

Area in hectares *2004*

- 100,000 or more
- 10,000 – 99,999
- 5,000 – 9,999
- 1,000 – 4,999
- less than 1,000
- no tobacco grown
- no data

tobacco grown on more than 1% of agricultural land *2002*

China
grew 37% of the world's tobacco in 2004.

Export value of tobacco
US$ millions
2003

World total: US$5,950,973

Brazil	$1,052.5
USA	$1,040.4
Zimbabwe	$464.6
Turkey	$329.0
Greece	$309.9
Italy	$293.5
Malawi	$290.4
Belgium	$236.7
China	$231.0
Germany	$185.0
India	$172.1

Cigarette manufacturing

Every year, more than 5 trillion cigarettes are manufactured worldwide. China is by far the largest cigarette manufacturer, followed by the USA.

The economic value of tobacco products amounts to hundreds of billions of US dollars per year. Very little goes to farmers for growing tobacco leaf. More is spent on paper, filters, and packaging than on tobacco. In the USA, the manufacturing sector's share of the tobacco dollar has almost tripled since 1970.

The tobacco industry has taken advantage of countries with inexpensive labour and a more friendly business environment to open new factories in Eastern Europe, for example. Technological advances in both farming and manufacturing are reducing the demand for manpower; this has a far greater impact on jobs than tobacco control efforts.

Cigarettes are highly engineered, exquisitely designed products, described by the US Food and Drug Administration as "nicotine delivery devices". Hundreds of chemicals are added to tobacco in the manufacture of cigarettes, making smoke easier to inhale and allowing companies to use less tobacco in each cigarette.

Aside from using less tobacco per cigarette, the composition of the cigarette is also changing. Manufacturers are increasingly using low-quality reconstituted tobacco because adding chemical additives is easier and making cigarettes from previously discarded plant parts, like leaf stems and tobacco dust, increases profit margins.

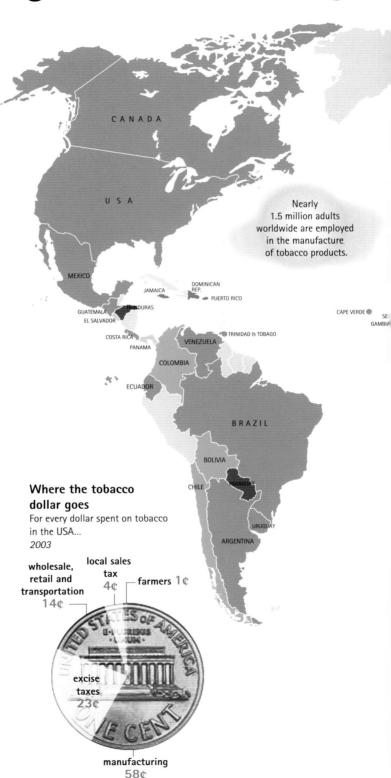

Nearly 1.5 million adults worldwide are employed in the manufacture of tobacco products.

Where the tobacco dollar goes

For every dollar spent on tobacco in the USA...
2003

wholesale, retail and transportation 14¢

local sales tax 4¢

farmers 1¢

excise taxes 23¢

manufacturing 58¢

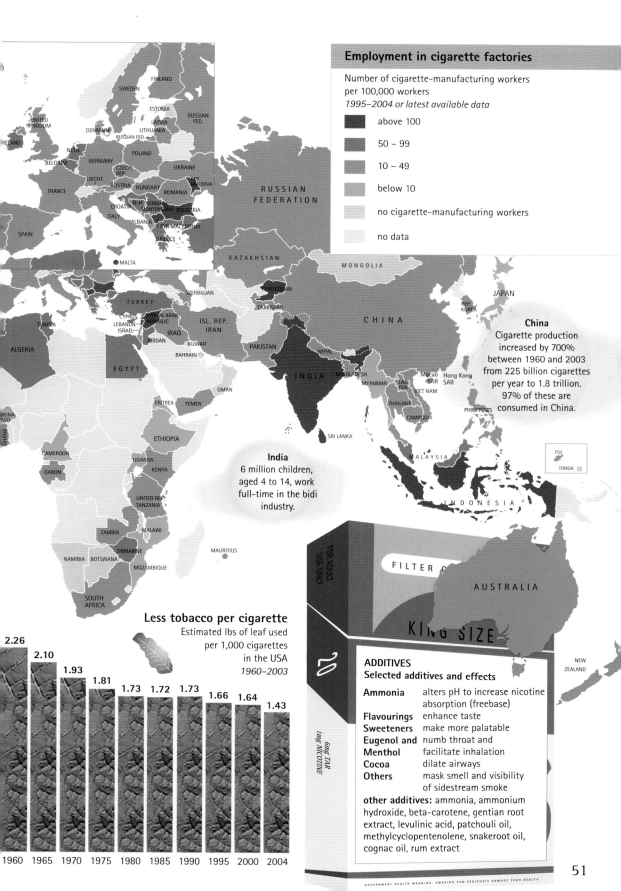

Employment in cigarette factories

Number of cigarette-manufacturing workers
per 100,000 workers
1995–2004 or latest available data

- above 100
- 50 – 99
- 10 – 49
- below 10
- no cigarette-manufacturing workers
- no data

China
Cigarette production
increased by 700%
between 1960 and 2003
from 225 billion cigarettes
per year to 1.8 trillion.
97% of these are
consumed in China.

India
6 million children,
aged 4 to 14, work
full-time in the bidi
industry.

Less tobacco per cigarette
Estimated lbs of leaf used
per 1,000 cigarettes
in the USA
1960–2003

1960	1965	1970	1975	1980	1985	1990	1995	2000	2004
2.26	2.10	1.93	1.81	1.73	1.72	1.73	1.66	1.64	1.43

FILTER

KING SIZE

FOR ADULT USE ONLY

20

6mg TAR
1mg NICOTINE

ADDITIVES
Selected additives and effects

Ammonia	alters pH to increase nicotine absorption (freebase)
Flavourings	enhance taste
Sweeteners	make more palatable
Eugenol and Menthol	numb throat and facilitate inhalation
Cocoa	dilate airways
Others	mask smell and visibility of sidestream smoke

other additives: ammonia, ammonium
hydroxide, beta-carotene, gentian root
extract, levulinic acid, patchouli oil,
methylcyclopentenolene, snakeroot oil,
cognac oil, rum extract

51

GOVERNMENT HEALTH WARNING: SMOKING CAN SERIOUSLY DAMAGE YOUR HEALTH

Tobacco companies

Altria Group, Inc, parent company of Philip Morris USA and Philip Morris International, is the largest transnational tobacco company and owner of the Marlboro brand, the world's top-selling cigarette since 1972. In 2004, Philip Morris captured about one-sixth of the world cigarette market by operating in 160 countries and selling cigarettes worth more than US$57 billion. British American Tobacco, the world's second-largest tobacco company, captured one-seventh of the global cigarette market in 2004 by selling 853 billion cigarettes under 300 brands in 180 markets.

The tobacco industry consists of a mixture of some of the most powerful transnational commercial companies in the world. Tobacco companies, which frequently merge, own other huge industries and run an intricate variety of joint-ventures. For instance, Japan Tobacco, half-owned by the Japanese government, markets Reynolds American cigarette brands (Camel, Salem and Winston) outside the USA, and owns food, beverage and pharmaceutical companies in Asia.

State tobacco monopolies have been in decline since the 1980s. Since the 1990s, the International Monetary Fund has pressured countries in Eastern Europe and Asia to privatize their state tobacco industry as a condition for loans. Since 2000, tobacco companies have gained access to state-owned markets in Colombia, Morocco and Romania.

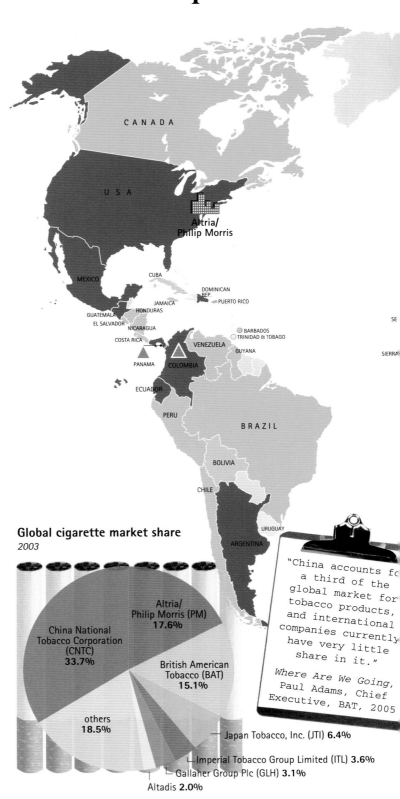

Global cigarette market share
2003

- China National Tobacco Corporation (CNTC) **33.7%**
- Altria/ Philip Morris (PM) **17.6%**
- British American Tobacco (BAT) **15.1%**
- others **18.5%**
- Japan Tobacco, Inc. (JTI) **6.4%**
- Imperial Tobacco Group Limited (ITL) **3.6%**
- Gallaher Group Plc (GLH) **3.1%**
- Altadis **2.0%**

"China accounts for a third of the global market for tobacco products, and international companies currently have very little share in it."

Where Are We Going, Paul Adams, Chief Executive, BAT, 2005

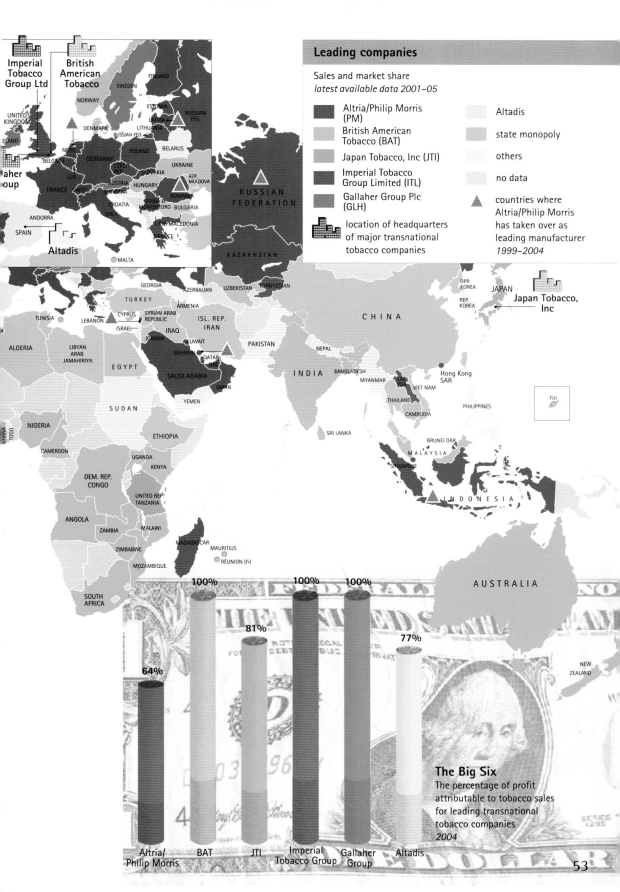

Leading companies

Sales and market share
latest available data 2001–05

- Altria/Philip Morris (PM)
- British American Tobacco (BAT)
- Japan Tobacco, Inc (JTI)
- Imperial Tobacco Group Limited (ITL)
- Gallaher Group Plc (GLH)
- Altadis
- state monopoly
- others
- no data

location of headquarters of major transnational tobacco companies

▲ countries where Altria/Philip Morris has taken over as leading manufacturer *1999–2004*

Imperial Tobacco Group Ltd

British American Tobacco

Japan Tobacco, Inc

Altadis

The Big Six
The percentage of profit attributable to tobacco sales for leading transnational tobacco companies *2004*

- Altria/Philip Morris — 64%
- BAT — 100%
- JTI — 81%
- Imperial Tobacco Group — 100%
- Gallaher Group — 100%
- Altadis — 77%

Tobacco trade

Tobacco trade is big business, for both the raw material (tobacco leaves) and the finished product (manufactured cigarettes). Brazil is the largest exporter of tobacco leaf and the Russian Federation is the largest importer.

Some countries that grow tobacco, such as the USA, export their own tobacco leaf while also importing foreign tobacco. Although the USA exports approximately the same amount of tobacco that it imports, the value of its leaf exports is double the value of imported leaf.

Political turmoil in Zimbabwe caused leaf production to collapse in the early 2000s, yet the global supply of tobacco leaf remained steady as production in Brazil and exports from China rose to meet demand. This indicates that supply-side controls are unlikely to limit the tobacco trade. Tobacco control requires measures that reduce demand.

In 2003, a total of 851 billion cigarettes were exported worldwide but only 664 billion cigarettes were reported as imports. The enormous number of "missing" cigarettes suggests that the global cigarette-smuggling problem could only continue with tobacco industry complicity.

"Despite the Asian financial crisis and the global economic slowdown, the potential of South-East Asia for the cigarette industry remains considerable."
Tobacco Reporter, 2002

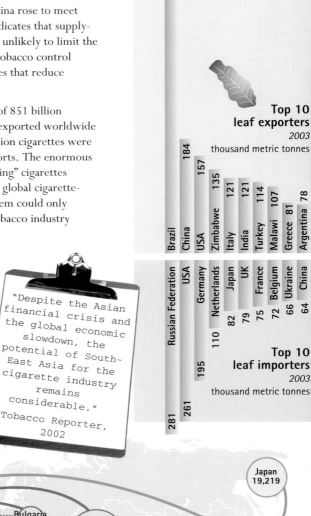

Top 10 leaf exporters
2003
thousand metric tonnes

Brazil	China	USA	Zimbabwe	Italy	India	Turkey	Malawi	Greece	Argentina
466	184	157	135	121	121	114	107	81	78

Top 10 leaf importers
2003
thousand metric tonnes

Russian Federation	USA	Germany	Netherlands	Japan	UK	France	Belgium	Ukraine	China
281	261	195	110	82	79	75	72	66	64

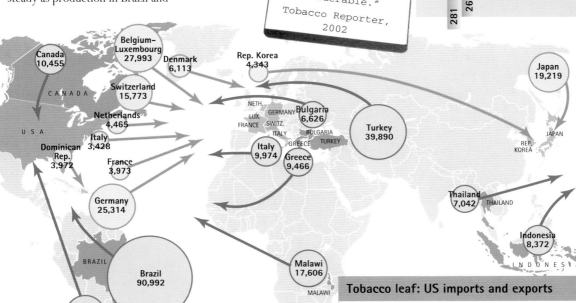

Canada 10,455 · Belgium–Luxembourg 27,993 · Denmark 6,113 · Rep. Korea 4,343 · Japan 19,219 · Switzerland 15,773 · Netherlands 4,465 · Italy 3,428 · France 3,973 · Dominican Rep. 3,972 · Germany 25,314 · Bulgaria 6,626 · Italy 9,974 · Greece 9,466 · Turkey 39,890 · Thailand 7,042 · Indonesia 8,372 · Brazil 90,992 · Malawi 17,606 · Argentina 18,685

Tobacco leaf: US imports and exports

2003 metric tonnes
total imported: 260,491
total exported: 155,448

↖ US imports
⟋ US exports

Cigarette exports

millions of cigarettes
2000–04

- over 100,000
- 10,000 – 99,999
- 5,000 – 9,999
- 1,000 – 4,999
- 100 – 999
- below 100
- do not export
- no data

Top 10 cigarette-importing countries
Number of cigarettes in billions
2003-04

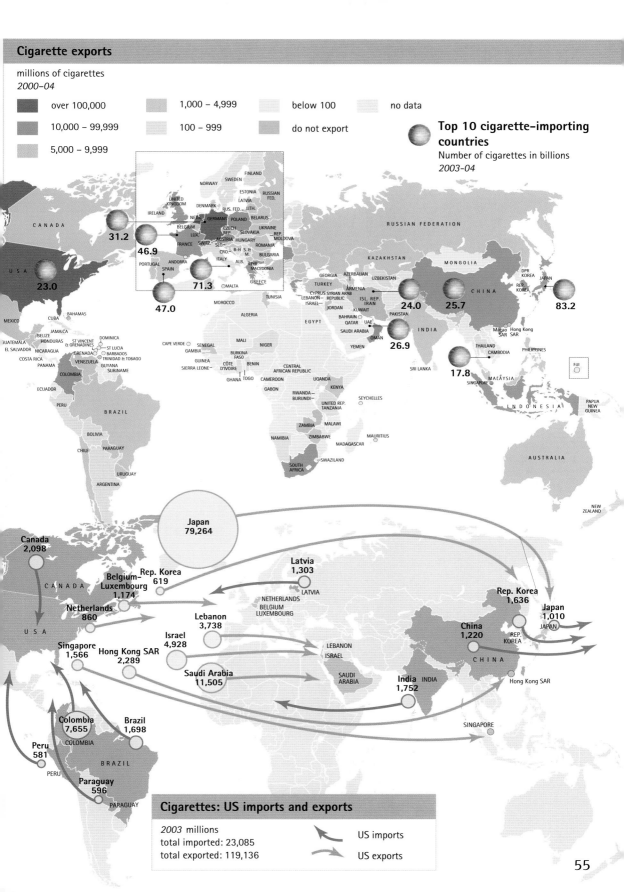

31.2
46.9
47.0
71.3
23.0
24.0
25.7
26.9
17.8
83.2

Japan 79,264

Canada 2,098

Belgium–Luxembourg 1,174
Rep. Korea 619
Netherlands 860
Latvia 1,303
Lebanon 3,738
Israel 4,928
Saudi Arabia 11,505
Singapore 1,566
Hong Kong SAR 2,289
Colombia 7,655
Brazil 1,698
Peru 581
Paraguay 596
China 1,220
Rep. Korea 1,636
Japan 1,010
India 1,752

Cigarettes: US imports and exports

2003 millions
total imported: 23,085
total exported: 119,136

↰ US imports
↱ US exports

55

Illegal cigarettes

Billions of cigarettes are smuggled each year, equal to about one-third of the total cigarette market. Cigarettes are the world's most widely smuggled legal consumer product. They are smuggled across almost every national border and along constantly changing routes.

Cigarette smuggling causes immeasurable harm. International brands become more affordable to low-income consumers and youth in developing countries, stimulating consumption. Tobacco companies reap greater profits while governments lose millions in tax revenue needed for tobacco control and to treat tobacco-related diseases. Cigarette smuggling bypasses legal restrictions and health regulations.

Smugglers are increasingly looking to counterfeit sources for their contraband. Between 2003 and 2004, 54 percent of seized cigarettes in the UK were counterfeit, three times more than between 2001 and 2002. The World Customs Organization estimates that China is a major source of "fake" cigarettes bound for sale in Europe with 190 billion counterfeit cigarettes produced each year.

Efforts to prevent cigarette smuggling are an important element of the WHO Framework Convention on Tobacco Control and international agreements to control smuggling are likely to be one of the first measures adopted.

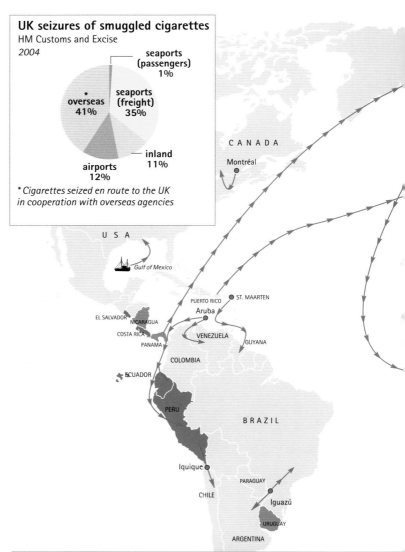

UK seizures of smuggled cigarettes
HM Customs and Excise
2004

- seaports (passengers) 1%
- seaports (freight) 35%
- *overseas 41%
- inland 11%
- airports 12%

Cigarettes seized en route to the UK in cooperation with overseas agencies

How to stop smuggling

The benefits of smuggling to the tobacco industry:
- no financial loss to industry, whereas governments lose tax revenue
- flooding of market with cheap cigarettes makes them more affordable to youth and encourages new smokers
- raises brand profile and promotes brand loyalty
- can use "smuggling argument" to dissuade governments from raising tobacco taxes
- gain access to markets closed to legitimate imports

Strategies to stop smuggling:
- monitor cigarette routes
- use technologically sophisticated "tax paid" markings on tobacco products identifying poi of origin and destination
- print unique serial numbers on all packages of tobacco products
- increase penalties
- collaborate with other countries via WHO FCTC and customs authorities

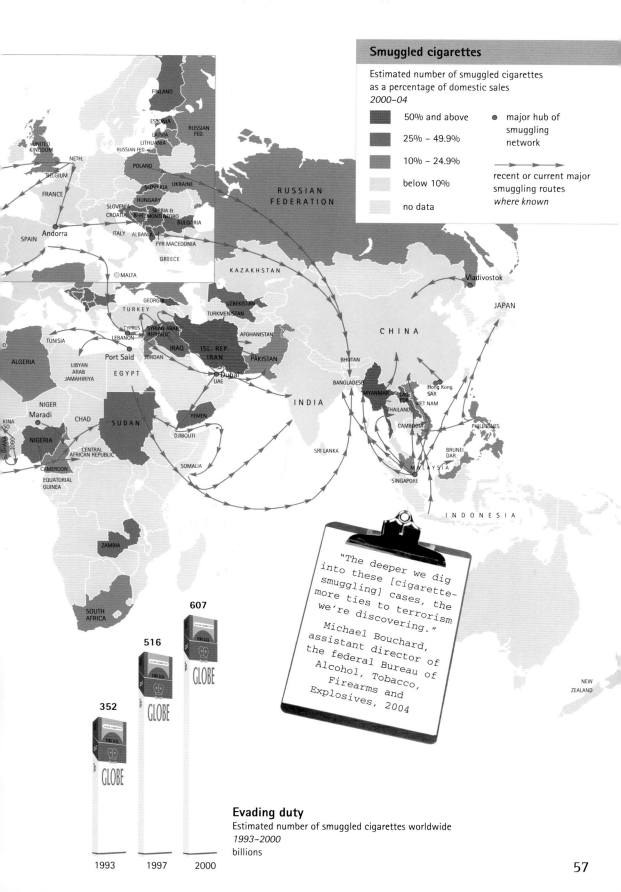

Estimated number of smuggled cigarettes
as a percentage of domestic sales
2000–04

50% and above	major hub of smuggling network
25% – 49.9%	
10% – 24.9%	recent or current major smuggling routes *where known*
below 10%	
no data	

FINLAND

ESTONIA
RUSSIAN FED.
LATVIA
LITHUANIA
RUSSIAN FED.

UNITED KINGDOM
NETH.
BELGIUM
POLAND
FRANCE
SLOVAKIA UKRAINE
HUNGARY
SLOVENIA
CROATIA SERBIA &
B–H MONTENEGRO
BULGARIA
Andorra
SPAIN ITALY ALBANIA
FYR MACEDONIA
GREECE
MALTA

RUSSIAN FEDERATION

KAZAKHSTAN

GEORGIA
TURKEY
UZBEKISTAN
TURKMENISTAN
CYPRUS
TUNISIA LEBANON SYRIAN ARAB REPUBLIC
AFGHANISTAN
ALGERIA JORDAN IRAQ ISL. REP. IRAN PAKISTAN
Port Said
LIBYAN ARAB JAMAHIRIYA
EGYPT Dubai
UAE
NIGER BHUTAN
Maradi CHAD BANGLADESH
KINA SO NIGERIA SUDAN YEMEN MYANMAR
GHANA TOGO CENTRAL AFRICAN REPUBLIC DJIBOUTI LAOS PDR
CAMEROON THAILAND
EQUATORIAL GUINEA SOMALIA CAMBODIA
SRI LANKA

CHINA
JAPAN
Vladivostok

INDIA
Hong Kong SAR
VIET NAM

PHILIPPINES
BRUNEI DAR.
MALAYSIA
SINGAPORE

ZAMBIA

SOUTH AFRICA

INDONESIA

NEW ZEALAND

> "The deeper we dig into these [cigarette-smuggling] cases, the more ties to terrorism we're discovering."
>
> Michael Bouchard, assistant director of the federal Bureau of Alcohol, Tobacco, Firearms and Explosives, 2004

607

516

352

Evading duty
Estimated number of smuggled cigarettes worldwide
1993–2000
billions

1993 1997 2000

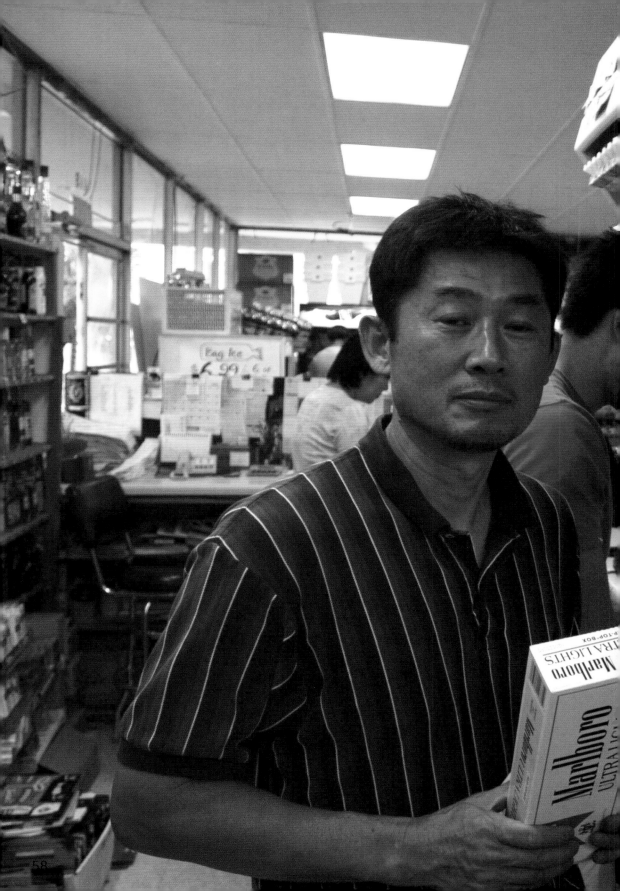

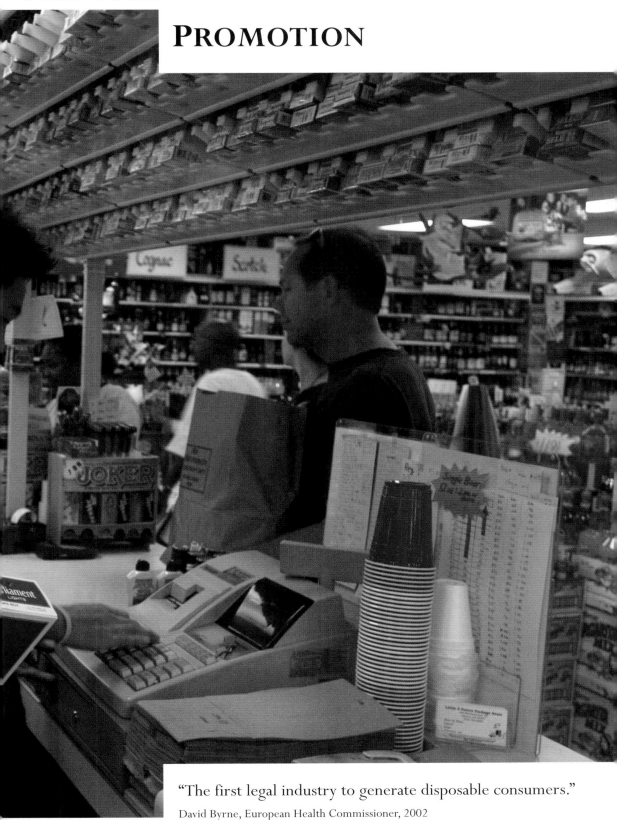

PART FOUR

PROMOTION

"The first legal industry to generate disposable consumers."

David Byrne, European Health Commissioner, 2002

"The pro-tobacco influence of the high smoking levels in recent movies will continue to be a pro-tobacco influence on teenagers for years to come unless remedial action is taken."
Professor Stan Glantz, University of California, San Francisco 2003

Tobacco companies compete fiercely for cigarette market share. Between 2000 and 2004, the top-selling brand changed in 20 percent of countries surveyed.

In the USA alone over US$15 billion is spent per year on marketing cigarettes. Annual marketing expenditures continue to rise despite falling cigarette sales and advertising bans on television, radio and at certain outdoor venues. Annual marketing expenditure amounts to about US$270 per smoker or 65 cents per pack. Price discounts – payments made to retailers to reduce the price of cigarettes to consumers – account for two-thirds of the total marketing expenditure.

Cigarette marketing is particularly bold and aggressive in many developing countries. Advertising on television and radio is common, and a variety of other venues are exploited, including sports, arts, music, street events, fashion, adventure tours, contests, giveaways and the internet.

Throughout both the developing and the developed world, subliminal advertising techniques are employed, such as the inclusion in films of gratuitous smoking behaviour and the strategic placement of cigarette brands.

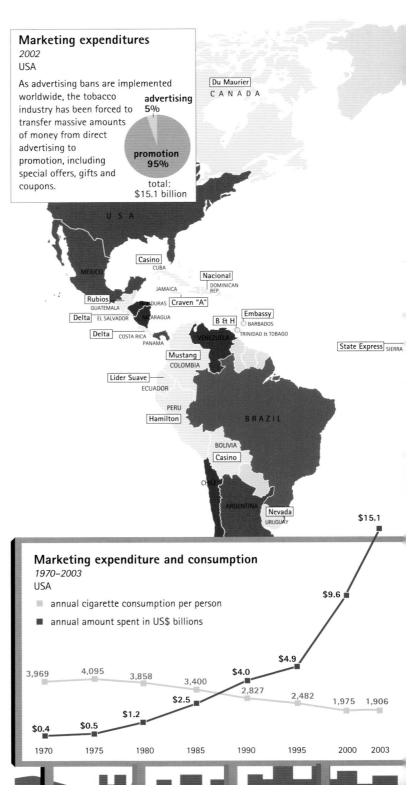

Marketing expenditures
2002
USA

As advertising bans are implemented worldwide, the tobacco industry has been forced to transfer massive amounts of money from direct advertising to promotion, including special offers, gifts and coupons.

advertising 5%
promotion 95%
total: $15.1 billion

Marketing expenditure and consumption
1970–2003
USA

□ annual cigarette consumption per person
■ annual amount spent in US$ billions

	1970	1975	1980	1985	1990	1995	2000	2003
consumption	3,969	4,095	3,858	3,400	2,827	2,482	1,975	1,906
spent	$0.4	$0.5	$1.2	$2.5	$4.0	$4.9	$9.6	$15.1

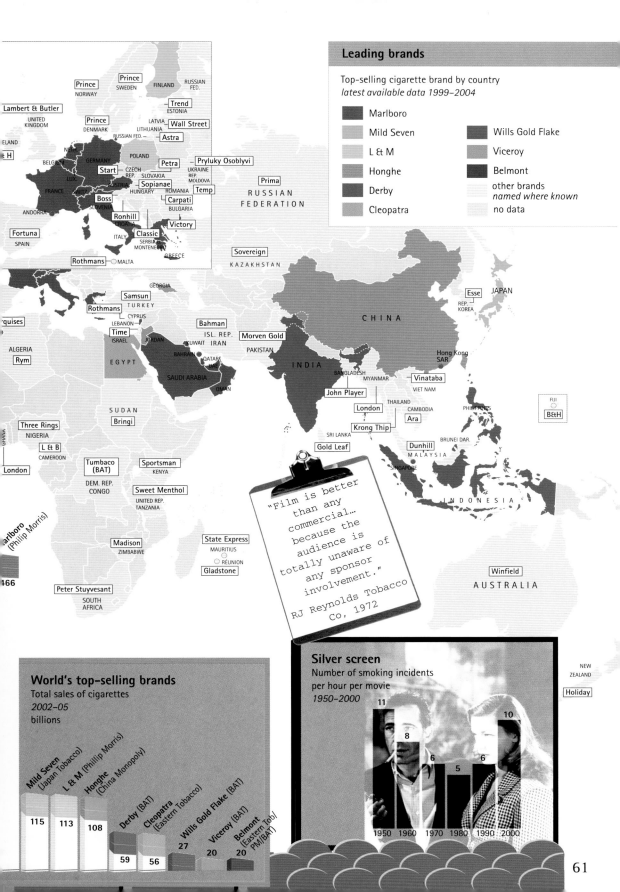

Leading brands

Top-selling cigarette brand by country
latest available data 1999–2004

- Marlboro
- Mild Seven
- L & M
- Honghe
- Derby
- Cleopatra
- Wills Gold Flake
- Viceroy
- Belmont
- other brands *named where known*
- no data

Map labels

Prince — NORWAY
Prince — SWEDEN
FINLAND
RUSSIAN FED.
Trend — ESTONIA
Lambert & Butler — UNITED KINGDOM
Prince — DENMARK
Wall Street — LATVIA
Astra — LITHUANIA
RUSSIAN FED.
& H
NETH
BELGIUM
LUX.
GERMANY
POLAND
Start — CZECH REP.
SLOVAKIA
Petra
Pryluky Osoblyvi — UKRAINE
REP. MOLDOVA
FRANCE
ANDORRA
SLOVENIA
Boss — AUSTRIA
HUNGARY
Sopianae
ROMANIA
Temp
Carpati
BULGARIA
Prima
Ronhill — CROATIA
Prima
RUSSIAN FEDERATION
ITALY
Classic — SERBIA MONTENEGRO
Victory
GREECE
Fortuna — SPAIN
Rothmans — MALTA
Sovereign
KAZAKHSTAN
quises
ALGERIA
Rym
GEORGIA
Samsun — TURKEY
Rothmans — CYPRUS
LEBANON
Esse — REP. KOREA
JAPAN
Time — ISRAEL
JORDAN
Bahman
ISL. REP. IRAN
Morven Gold — PAKISTAN
CHINA
Hong Kong SAR
KUWAIT
BAHRAIN
QATAR
SAUDI ARABIA
OMAN
EGYPT
INDIA
BANGLADESH
MYANMAR
Vinataba — VIET NAM
FUJI
B&H
SUDAN
Bringi
John Player
THAILAND
CAMBODIA
Ara
London
PHILIPPINES
Three Rings — NIGERIA
L & B — CAMEROON
London
Krong Thip
SRI LANKA
Gold Leaf
Dunhill — MALAYSIA
BRUNEI DAR.
SINGAPORE
Tumbaco (BAT) — DEM. REP. CONGO
Sportsman — KENYA
Sweet Menthol — UNITED REP. TANZANIA
INDONESIA
Madison — ZIMBABWE
State Express — MAURITIUS
RÉUNION
Gladstone
Winfield
AUSTRALIA
Marlboro (Philip Morris)
466
Peter Stuyvesant — SOUTH AFRICA
NEW ZEALAND
Holiday

"Film is better than any commercial… because the audience is totally unaware of any sponsor involvement."
RJ Reynolds Tobacco Co, 1972

World's top-selling brands

Total sales of cigarettes
2002–05
billions

- Mild Seven (Japan Tobacco) — 115
- L & M (Phillip Morris) — 113
- Honghe (China Monopoly) — 108
- Derby (BAT) — 59
- Cleopatra (Eastern Tobacco) — 56
- Wills Gold Flake (BAT) — 27
- Viceroy (BAT) — 20
- Belmont (Eastern Tob/ PM/BAT) — 20

Silver screen

Number of smoking incidents per hour per movie
1950–2000

1950	1960	1970	1980	1990	2000
11	8	6	5	6	10

Buying influence

"The tobacco industry continues to wield enormous political influence by spending millions on campaign contributions and lobbyists' salaries. It is disappointing that once again Congress has failed to put the interests of the public's health before Big Tobacco's agenda."
Chellie Pingree,
Common Cause President, 2004

"Political will to promote public health and a strong tobacco control advocacy presence can enable governments to resist the enormous pressure exerted upon them by multinational tobacco companies."
J Knight and S Chapman,
University of Sydney, Australia 2004

The tobacco industry spends tens of millions of dollars to influence public policy. Tobacco companies make major cash contributions to elected officials and political parties, subsidize air travel, finance political conventions and inaugurations, and host fundraisers

for politicians. Tobacco companies also donate a small percentage of their profits to civic, educational and charitable organizations to enhance their public image.

Tobacco companies conduct direct lobbying and sophisticated public relations campaigns using paid media to influence the opinions of political decision-makers.

For instance, the tobacco industry spent nearly $10.4 million to lobby the United States Congress in the first six months of 2004. That amounts to about $122,000 for every day Congress was in session.

A bill introducing comprehensive tobacco control legislation was defeated in the US Senate in 1998.

Senators who voted against the legislation had received, on average, nearly four times more money from the tobacco industry in the two years before their last election than those who voted in favour of the bill.

Tobacco industry tactics have been extended to countries throughout the world. Buying influence and favours through political contributions is common practice; however, most countries do not require mandatory reporting of tobacco industry inducements. The tobacco industry continues to promote its agenda using deceptive "front" organizations, such as "smoker's alliances" and industry-funded international consortiums.

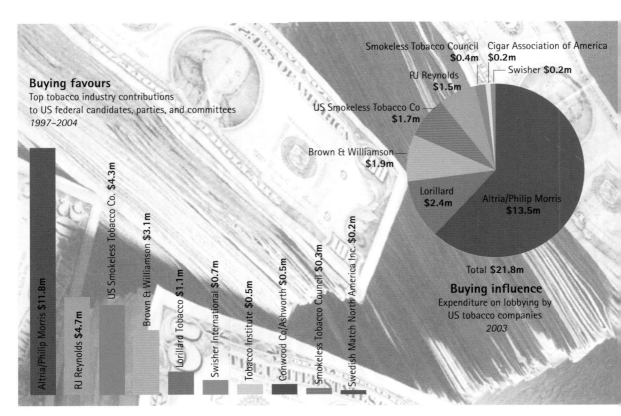

Buying favours
Top tobacco industry contributions to US federal candidates, parties, and committees
1997–2004

Altria/Philip Morris $11.8m
RJ Reynolds $4.7m
US Smokeless Tobacco Co. $4.3m
Brown & Williamson $3.1m
Lorillard Tobacco $1.1m
Swisher International $0.7m
Tobacco Institute $0.5m
Conwood Co/Ashworth $0.5m
Smokeless Tobacco Council $0.3m
Swedish Match North America Inc. $0.2m

Smokeless Tobacco Council $0.4m   Cigar Association of America $0.2m
RJ Reynolds $1.5m   Swisher $0.2m
US Smokeless Tobacco Co $1.7m
Brown & Williamson $1.9m
Lorillard $2.4m
Altria/Philip Morris $13.5m

Total $21.8m
Buying influence
Expenditure on lobbying by
US tobacco companies
2003

"Small shopkeepers were enlisted to write protests to members of Parliament; the letters 'some with deliberate typographical errors to create the aura of authenticity,' were prepared by the (tobacco) industry for the shopkeepers."

Philip Morris, 1990

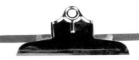

"We have got the unions to support industry in several countries. Prominent have been the efforts they have made on the tax issues in the UK where they were very involved in a letter writing campaign to Members of Parliament."

Philip Morris, 1985

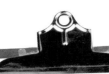

"Aside from delaying the adoption of a convention the company is best served by participating in the development of the agreement. It would be in the company's interest to have the treaty focus entirely on protecting children and leaving adult choice protected…"

Jack Mongoven, 1997, of Mongoven, Biscoe, and Duchin (MBD), a specialist firm hired by Philip Morris to analyze the WHO FCTC process.

"Turning now to primary and passive smoking…To get more favorable press, we are contemplating organizing another journalists' conference similar to the one we put together in Madrid for Latin American journalists in 1984."

Philip Morris, 1985

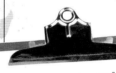

"Philip Morris and the industry are positively impacting the government decisions of Bahrain, Kuwait, Oman, Qatar, Saudi Arabia and the UAE through the creative use of market specific studies, position papers, well briefed distributors who lobby, media owners and consultants…"

Philip Morris, 1987

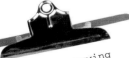

"What are we trying to accomplish? Prevent further deterioration of overall social, legislative and regulatory climate, and ultimately, actually improve the climate for the marketing and use of tobacco products."

Philip Morris, 1990

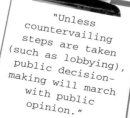

"Unless countervailing steps are taken (such as lobbying), public decision-making will march with public opinion."

RJ Reynolds, 1978

Tobacco industry documents

"On May 12, 1994, an unsolicited box of what appeared to be tobacco company documents was delivered to Professor Stanton Glantz at the University of California, San Francisco (UCSF). The documents in the box dated from the early 1950s to the early 1980s. They consisted primarily of confidential internal memoranda related to B&W and BAT. Many of the documents contained internal discussions of the tobacco industry's public relations and legal strategies over the years, and they were often labelled 'confidential' or 'privileged'. The return address on the box was simply 'Mr Butts'."

So begins *The Cigarette Papers*, the first report chronicling the release of previously secret tobacco industry documents. Public release of these documents clearly illustrated their power in exposing tobacco industry corporate behaviour, and they profoundly influenced public opinion.

Following the release of the BAT documents and as a result of litigation and legal settlement agreements in the USA, documents introduced through legal discovery have had to be made publicly available by the tobacco industry in physical depositories in Minnesota, USA and Guildford, UK. Subsequent rulings released the "Bliley Documents", approximately 32,000 records censored from industry sites because the companies continue to claim that they are privileged and confidential. Today, documents in the BAT Guildford Depository are available to tobacco control researchers via the internet.

"The continuing challenge for tobacco control advocates is how to search through these documents, find the most relevant documents for legislative and regulatory efforts and then use them to good effect."
Framework Convention Alliance, 2005

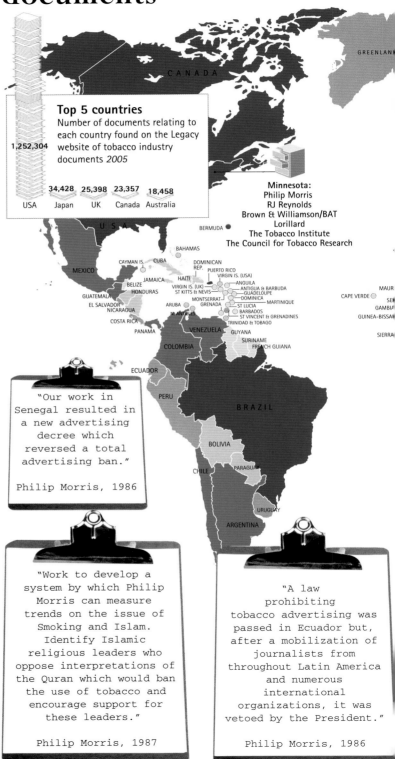

Top 5 countries
Number of documents relating to each country found on the Legacy website of tobacco industry documents *2005*

1,252,304

USA	Japan	UK	Canada	Australia
34,428	25,398	23,357	18,458	

Minnesota:
Philip Morris
RJ Reynolds
Brown & Williamson/BAT
Lorillard
The Tobacco Institute
The Council for Tobacco Research

"Our work in Senegal resulted in a new advertising decree which reversed a total advertising ban."

Philip Morris, 1986

"Work to develop a system by which Philip Morris can measure trends on the issue of Smoking and Islam. Identify Islamic religious leaders who oppose interpretations of the Quran which would ban the use of tobacco and encourage support for these leaders."

Philip Morris, 1987

"A law prohibiting tobacco advertising was passed in Ecuador but, after a mobilization of journalists from throughout Latin America and numerous international organizations, it was vetoed by the President."

Philip Morris, 1986

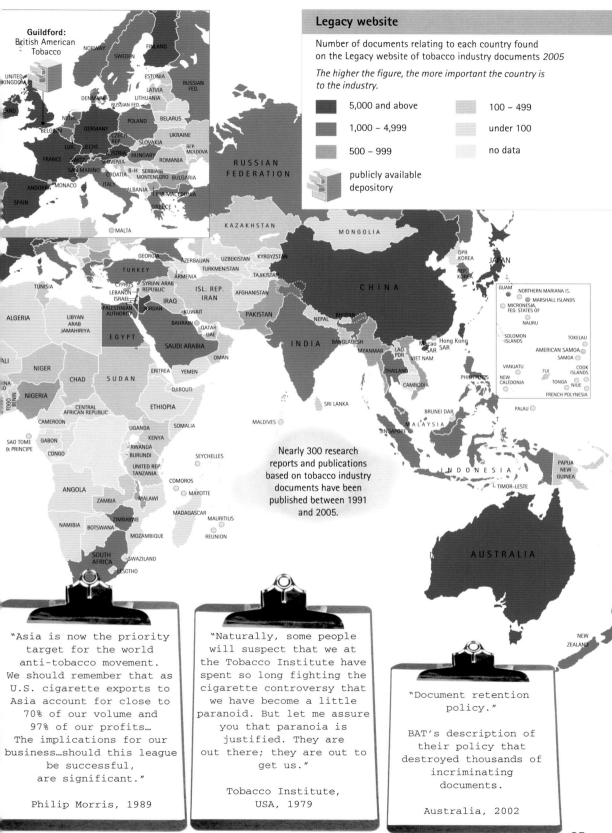

Legacy website

Number of documents relating to each country found on the Legacy website of tobacco industry documents 2005

The higher the figure, the more important the country is to the industry.

- 5,000 and above
- 1,000 – 4,999
- 500 – 999
- 100 – 499
- under 100
- no data
- publicly available depository

Guildford: British American Tobacco

Nearly 300 research reports and publications based on tobacco industry documents have been published between 1991 and 2005.

"Asia is now the priority target for the world anti-tobacco movement. We should remember that as U.S. cigarette exports to Asia account for close to 70% of our volume and 97% of our profits… The implications for our business…should this league be successful, are significant."

Philip Morris, 1989

"Naturally, some people will suspect that we at the Tobacco Institute have spent so long fighting the cigarette controversy that we have become a little paranoid. But let me assure you that paranoia is justified. They are out there; they are out to get us."

Tobacco Institute, USA, 1979

"Document retention policy."

BAT's description of their policy that destroyed thousands of incriminating documents.

Australia, 2002

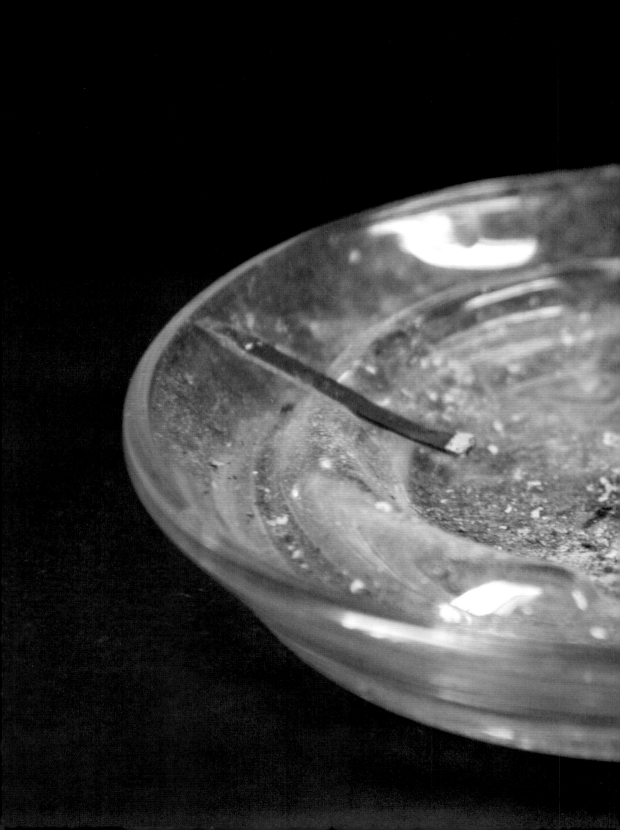

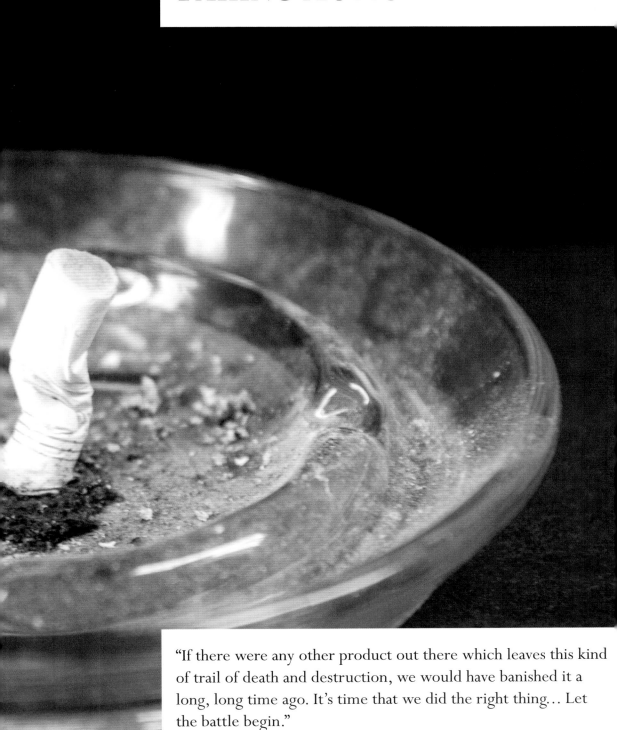

PART FIVE

TAKING ACTION

"If there were any other product out there which leaves this kind of trail of death and destruction, we would have banished it a long, long time ago. It's time that we did the right thing… Let the battle begin."

George Smitherman, Minister of Health and Long-Term Care for Ontario, Ontario Tobacco Control Conference, 2004

Research

Since the 1950s, scientific research has proven the extensive harm tobacco causes to human health.

Scientific evidence from developed countries and an increasing number of developing countries has accumulated on tobacco use, the harm it causes, and actions needed to discourage its use. Barriers that make it difficult for developing countries to participate in tobacco control research stem mainly from insufficient investment in the infrastructure for health sciences research. This results in a lack of standardized data on tobacco consumption, weak communication networks, and a shortage of health research professionals.

To improve their public image, tobacco companies offer substantial research funding to academic institutions worldwide. Accepting donations from tobacco companies is controversial within the academic community and many institutions prohibit it to protect the integrity of their research. Too often, tobacco companies have sponsored academic research, assuring complete independence, only to suppress unfavourable findings. Alternatively, findings that support the tobacco industry have been published without proper disclosure of the sponsor's role in the research.

In addition to financial disclosure, researchers who publish in medical journals should explicitly describe the extent of the tobacco industry's role in designing, conducting, and reporting results of a study.

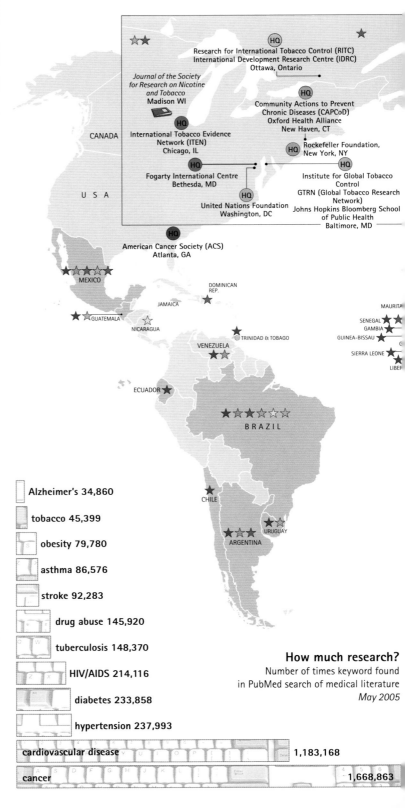

How much research?
Number of times keyword found in PubMed search of medical literature
May 2005

Alzheimer's 34,860

tobacco 45,399

obesity 79,780

asthma 86,576

stroke 92,283

drug abuse 145,920

tuberculosis 148,370

HIV/AIDS 214,116

diabetes 233,858

hypertension 237,993

cardiovascular disease 1,183,168

cancer 1,668,863

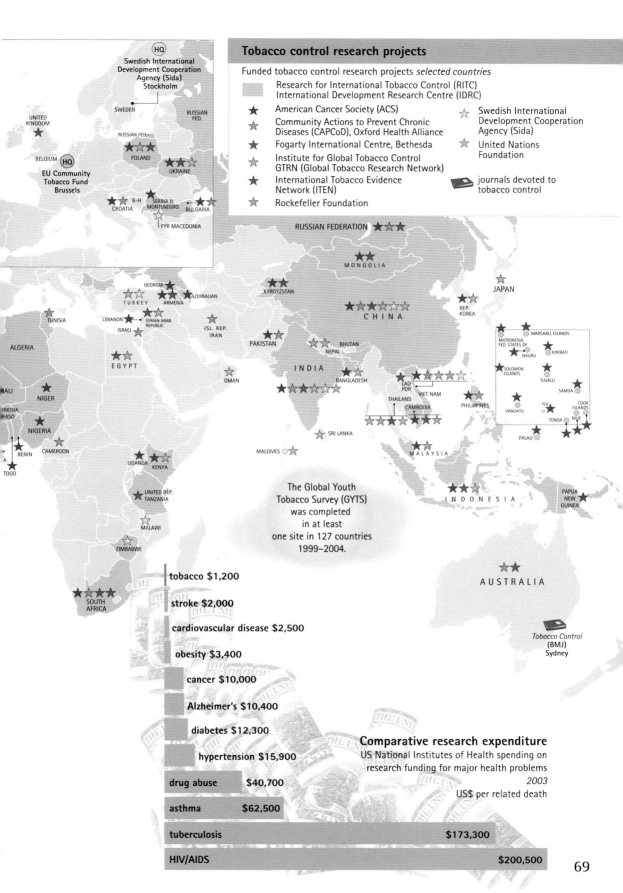

Tobacco control research projects

Funded tobacco control research projects *selected countries*

Research for International Tobacco Control (RITC)
International Development Research Centre (IDRC)

★ American Cancer Society (ACS)

★ Community Actions to Prevent Chronic Diseases (CAPCoD), Oxford Health Alliance

★ Fogarty International Centre, Bethesda

☆ Institute for Global Tobacco Control
GTRN (Global Tobacco Research Network)

★ International Tobacco Evidence Network (ITEN)

☆ Rockefeller Foundation

☆ Swedish International Development Cooperation Agency (Sida)

☆ United Nations Foundation

📔 journals devoted to tobacco control

Swedish International Development Cooperation Agency (Sida) Stockholm

EU Community Tobacco Fund Brussels

The Global Youth Tobacco Survey (GYTS) was completed in at least one site in 127 countries 1999–2004.

Tobacco Control (BMJ) Sydney

Comparative research expenditure
US National Institutes of Health spending on research funding for major health problems
2003
US$ per related death

tobacco $1,200
stroke $2,000
cardiovascular disease $2,500
obesity $3,400
cancer $10,000
Alzheimer's $10,400
diabetes $12,300
hypertension $15,900
drug abuse $40,700
asthma $62,500
tuberculosis $173,300
HIV/AIDS $200,500

"While the WHO FCTC provides the framework for action against tobacco, the actual work to combat tobacco use must necessarily occur at country level. The success of the WHO FCTC will depend almost entirely on the ability of countries to implement and enforce its provisions."
Dr Lee Jong-wook, Director-General, WHO, 2005

The United Nations Development Programme defines capacity as "the ability to perform functions, solve problems and achieve objectives" at three levels: individual, institutional and societal." National capacity building is at the forefront of tobacco control initiatives. Since the adoption of WHO's Framework Convention on Tobacco Control in 2003, many countries, especially those in the developing world, face the challenge of developing national plans of action, often without the expertise, leadership or data gathering and surveillance infrastructures. Thus, capacity-building programmes focus on enhancing these elements.

The Framework Convention Alliance (FCA), an umbrella organization of 200 tobacco control organizations, contributes significantly to capacity-building efforts in 80 countries around the world by organizing workshops and providing technical expertise in support of ratification and implementation of the WHO FCTC.

Many organizations work to enhance national capacity-building efforts by facilitating international research communication and collaboration, managing, and disseminating information on the health hazards, economic damage, and environmental costs of tobacco use.

GLOBALink, an internet-based network of tobacco control advocates from around the world, is one of the most important resources available for capacity building. Activists and advocates continuously share their knowledge and experience on a broad range of public health, medical, legal, technical, social and cultural issues related to tobacco control through the GLOBALink network.

Through the unified and coordinated efforts of thousands of dedicated individuals, the Herculean task of global tobacco control is becoming a reality.

Additional organizations 2005

- Action on Smoking and Health, USA
- Cancer Research UK
- Cancer Council Australia
- Framework Convention Alliance for Tobacco Control
- French Cancer League
- Global Tobacco Research Network
- International Union for Health Promotion and Education
- Norwegian Cancer Society
- Open Society Institute
- Program for Appropriate Technology in Health (PATH Canada)
- Swedish International Development Agency

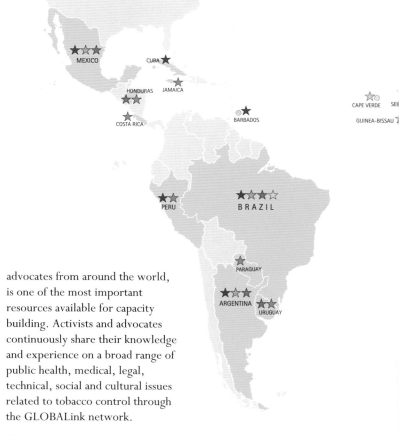

Plans of action

Organizations funding capacity-building projects
2005

countries that participate in, are funded for, or implement capacity-building projects

★ 11th World Conference on Tobacco or Health

☆ American Cancer Society/International Union Against Cancer

★ American Cancer Society/International Union Against Cancer/Cancer Research UK

★ American Cancer Society/Research for International Tobacco Control/Canadian Tobacco Control Research Initiative

☆ Romania Tobacco Control

★ Tobacco Free Initiative

☆ other

RUSSIAN FED.

RUSSIAN FED. — LITHUANIA

POLAND

CZECH REP. SLOVAKIA UKRAINE

HUNGARY ROMANIA

CROATIA

SERBIA & MONTENEGRO BULGARIA

RUSSIAN FEDERATION

KAZAKHSTAN

MONGOLIA

GEORGIA

ARMENIA UZBEKISTAN KYRGYZSTAN

TUNISIA

ALGERIA

ISL. REP. IRAN

JORDAN

PAKISTAN NEPAL

CHINA

REP. KOREA

UAE

INDIA BANGLADESH

MYANMAR LAO PDR VIET NAM

THAILAND

MICRONESIA, FED. STATES OF

MARSHALL ISLANDS

NAURU KIRIBATI

SOLOMON ISLANDS TUVALU

SAMOA

VANUATU FIJI COOK NIUE IS.

TONGA

NIGER CHAD SUDAN YEMEN

DJIBOUTI

KINA SO

TOGO BENIN NIGERIA

CAMEROON

UGANDA KENYA

SAO TOME & PRINCIPE GABON SOMALIA

ANA

DEM. REP. CONGO UNITED REP. TANZANIA

COMOROS

ANGOLA ZAMBIA MALAWI

MADAGASCAR MAURITIUS

BOTSWANA MOZAMBIQUE

MALAYSIA

PHILIPPINES

PALAU

PAPUA NEW GUINEA

L TIMOR-LESTE

Key strategies to strengthen national capacity for tobacco control

- Analyse the national tobacco control situation
- Develop consensus and political commitment
- Outline national tobacco control strategies
- Establish a national co-ordination committee
- Build a comprehensive national plan of action
- Establish sustained funding mechanisms
- Incorporate national tobacco control efforts into existing health structures to ensure sustainability
- Develop strategies for monitoring and counteraction of tobacco industry activities in rural areas
- Establish a system of monitoring and evaluating tobacco control policies, development and implementation

Framework Convention on Tobacco Control

"Expect a convention to please no-one, but hope it will be acceptable to everyone."
Paul Szasz, UN expert on international law, on the WHO FCTC, 2002

Out of 192 WHO Member States and the European Community, 167 have signed the WHO FCTC. It came into effect on 27 February 2005, making it one of the most rapidly embraced international treaties of all time.

The treaty helps legislators realize that the tide of tobacco control is international and unstoppable, good for both the wealth and health of nations. It will make it more difficult for the tobacco industry to derail future tobacco control legislation.

Not surprisingly, the tobacco industry was against a strong, legally binding FCTC, and sought voluntary agreements and self-regulating market mechanisms, which are essentially ineffective.

The tobacco industry need not fear the FCTC, as between 2005 and 2025 the number of smokers worldwide is predicted to rise from 1.3 billion smokers to 1.5 billion, mainly due to population increase, assuming a global annual reduction in prevalence of 1 percent. Analysis by health economists concluded that the FCTC will not harm national economies, even of tobacco growing nations, especially as the FCTC deals primarily with demand reduction strategies, except for the control of smuggling. Already the treaty has mobilized resources; rallied hundreds of non-governmental organizations (NGOs); encouraged government action; led to the political maturation of health ministries; and raised awareness among other government ministries.

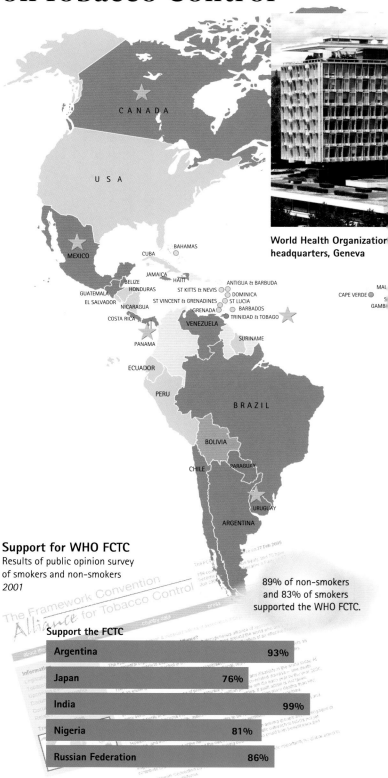

World Health Organization headquarters, Geneva

Support for WHO FCTC

Results of public opinion survey of smokers and non-smokers
2001

89% of non-smokers and 83% of smokers supported the WHO FCTC.

Support the FCTC

Argentina	93%
Japan	76%
India	99%
Nigeria	81%
Russian Federation	86%

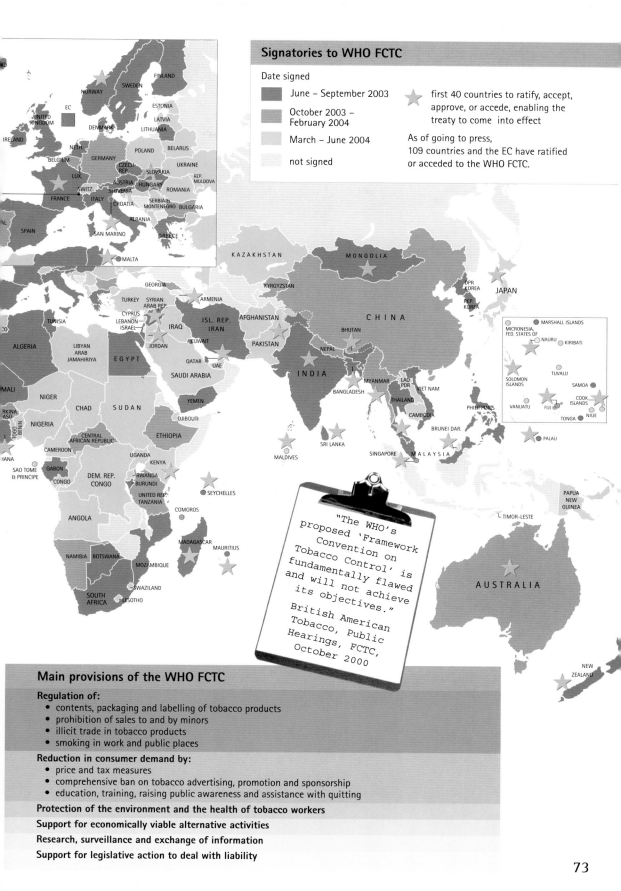

Date signed

June – September 2003

October 2003 – February 2004

March – June 2004

not signed

first 40 countries to ratify, accept, approve, or accede, enabling the treaty to come into effect

As of going to press, 109 countries and the EC have ratified or acceded to the WHO FCTC.

"The WHO's proposed 'Framework Convention on Tobacco Control' is fundamentally flawed and will not achieve its objectives."

British American Tobacco, Public Hearings, FCTC, October 2000

Main provisions of the WHO FCTC

Regulation of:
- contents, packaging and labelling of tobacco products
- prohibition of sales to and by minors
- illicit trade in tobacco products
- smoking in work and public places

Reduction in consumer demand by:
- price and tax measures
- comprehensive ban on tobacco advertising, promotion and sponsorship
- education, training, raising public awareness and assistance with quitting

Protection of the environment and the health of tobacco workers

Support for economically viable alternative activities

Research, surveillance and exchange of information

Support for legislative action to deal with liability

"Fears in the hospitality industry that smoking bans may damage business interests are largely unfounded." World Bank, 2002

There is no safe level of exposure to environmental tobacco smoke.

Smoking bans benefit non-smokers and smokers alike. Non-smokers are exposed to significantly less second-hand smoke, while smokers tend to smoke less, have greater cessation success, and increased confidence in their ability to quit. These effects are more significant under a full ban than under a partial one. When indoor smoking areas are allowed, ventilation is inadequate to eliminate second-hand smoke and the reduction in smoking among smokers is less significant.

Smoking bans are economically beneficial to employers. Smoking bans are relatively inexpensive to implement, and lead to a reduction in accidental fires, lower insurance premiums, and reduced employee absenteeism.

Support is growing for smoking bans in public places. In many countries with little or no legislation on smoke-free areas, the public is overwhelmingly in favour of bans being put into place. In many areas where smoking bans are mandated by law, employees, customers, and business owners report satisfaction with the results.

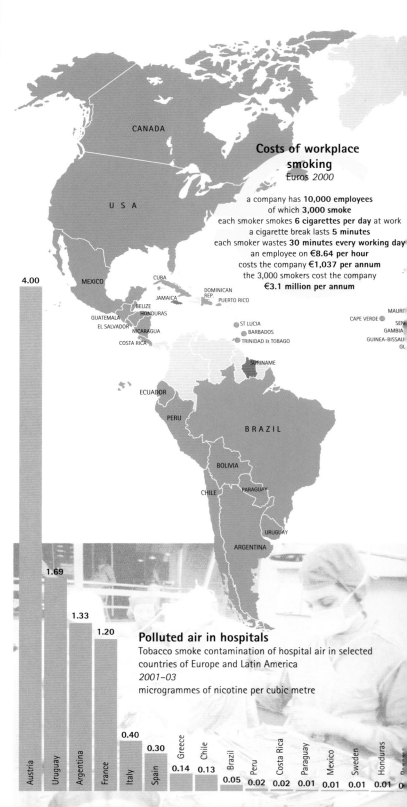

Costs of workplace smoking
Euros 2000

a company has **10,000 employees** of which **3,000 smoke** each smoker smokes **6 cigarettes per day** at work a cigarette break lasts **5 minutes** each smoker wastes **30 minutes every working day** an employee on **€8.64 per hour** costs the company **€1,037 per annum** the 3,000 smokers cost the company **€3.1 million per annum**

Polluted air in hospitals
Tobacco smoke contamination of hospital air in selected countries of Europe and Latin America
2001–03
microgrammes of nicotine per cubic metre

Austria	4.00
Uruguay	1.69
Argentina	1.33
France	1.20
Italy	0.40
Spain	0.30
Greece	0.14
Chile	0.13
Brazil	0.05
Peru	0.02
Costa Rica	0.02
Paraguay	0.01
Mexico	0.01
Sweden	0.01
Honduras	0.01

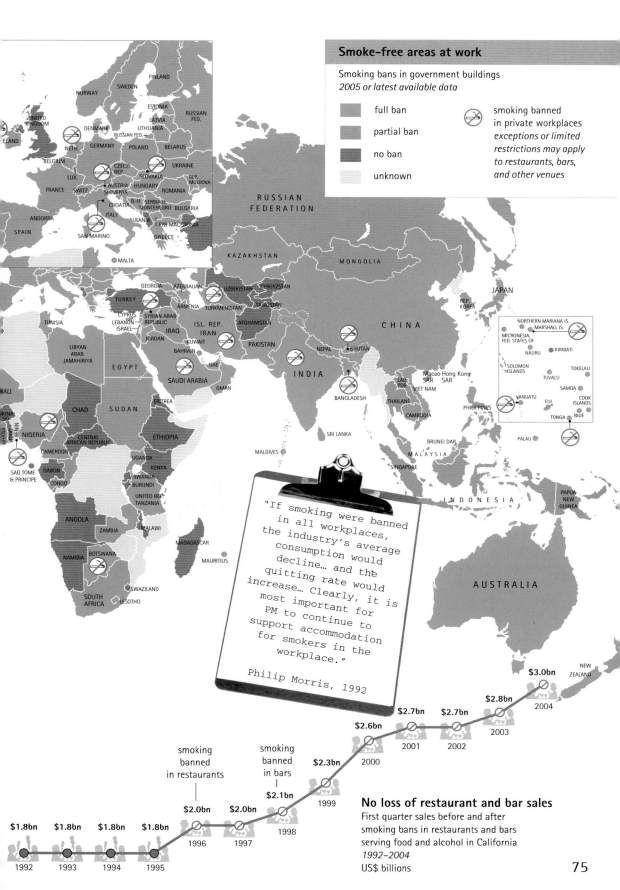

Smoke-free areas at work

Smoking bans in government buildings
2005 or latest available data

- full ban
- partial ban
- no ban
- unknown

🚭 smoking banned
in private workplaces
*exceptions or limited
restrictions may apply
to restaurants, bars,
and other venues*

Map labels:
FINLAND, SWEDEN, NORWAY, ESTONIA, RUSSIAN FED., LATVIA, LITHUANIA, UNITED KINGDOM, DENMARK, RUSSIAN FED., IRELAND, GERMANY, POLAND, BELARUS, NETH., BELGIUM, CZECH REP., UKRAINE, LUX., SLOVAKIA, FRANCE, SWITZ., AUSTRIA, HUNGARY, REP. MOLDOVA, SLOVENIA, ROMANIA, ANDORRA, CROATIA, B-H, SERBIA & MONTENEGRO, BULGARIA, SPAIN, ITALY, ALBANIA, FYR MACEDONIA, SAN MARINO, GREECE, MALTA

RUSSIAN FEDERATION, KAZAKHSTAN, MONGOLIA, JAPAN

TUNISIA, TURKEY, GEORGIA, AZERBAIJAN, KYRGYZSTAN, UZBEKISTAN, REP. KOREA, CYPRUS, ARMENIA, TURKMENISTAN, TAJIKISTAN, LEBANON, SYRIAN ARAB REPUBLIC, ISRAEL, IRAQ, ISL. REP. IRAN, AFGHANISTAN, CHINA, JORDAN, KUWAIT, LIBYAN ARAB JAMAHIRIYA, BAHRAIN, PAKISTAN, NEPAL, BHUTAN, EGYPT, UAE, SAUDI ARABIA, OMAN, INDIA, NEPAL, BANGLADESH, LAO PDR, VIET NAM, MACAO, HONG KONG SAR, MALI, CHAD, SUDAN, ERITREA, THAILAND, CAMBODIA, PHILIPPINES, BURKINA FASO, CENTRAL AFRICAN REPUBLIC, ETHIOPIA, SRI LANKA, BRUNEI DAR, NIGERIA, BENIN, TOGO, CAMEROON, UGANDA, KENYA, MALDIVES, MALAYSIA, SINGAPORE, SAO TOME & PRINCIPE, GABON, CONGO, RWANDA, BURUNDI, UNITED REP. TANZANIA, INDONESIA, PAPUA NEW GUINEA, ANGOLA, ZAMBIA, MALAWI, MADAGASCAR, MAURITIUS, NAMIBIA, BOTSWANA, AUSTRALIA, SWAZILAND, SOUTH AFRICA, LESOTHO, NEW ZEALAND

NORTHERN MARIANA IS., MARSHALL IS., MICRONESIA, FED. STATES OF, NAURU, KIRIBATI, SOLOMON ISLANDS, TOKELAU, TUVALU, VANUATU, FIJI, SAMOA, COOK ISLANDS, TONGA, NIUE, PALAU

Quote on clipboard:
"If smoking were banned in all workplaces, the industry's average consumption would decline… and the quitting rate would increase… Clearly, it is most important for PM to continue to support accommodation for smokers in the workplace."

Philip Morris, 1992

No loss of restaurant and bar sales

First quarter sales before and after smoking bans in restaurants and bars serving food and alcohol in California
1992–2004
US$ billions

- 1992 — $1.8bn
- 1993 — $1.8bn
- 1994 — $1.8bn
- 1995 — $1.8bn
- 1996 — $2.0bn | smoking banned in restaurants
- 1997 — $2.0bn
- 1998 — $2.1bn | smoking banned in bars
- 1999 — $2.3bn
- 2000 — $2.6bn
- 2001 — $2.7bn
- 2002 — $2.7bn
- 2003 — $2.8bn
- 2004 — $3.0bn

"Advertising is a valuable economic factor because it is the cheapest way of selling goods, particularly if the goods are worthless."
Sinclair Lewis, American novelist and playwright (1885–1951)

Tobacco product marketing encourages people to start smoking and increases the amount smoked. Recognizing the impact of such marketing, many countries have imposed restrictions on tobacco marketing. However, research shows that partial restrictions are ineffective in reducing smoking because tobacco companies simply redirect their marketing efforts to other available venues. Only comprehensive bans on all forms of tobacco advertising, marketing, and promotion are effective at reducing smoking rates.

In the face of growing restrictions and bans on tobacco marketing, tobacco companies have become increasingly creative in their attempts to sustain a market for their product. Brand stretching, event promotion, retailer incentives, and advertising in international media are some of the ways that the tobacco industry circumvents advertising bans.

Cigarette packets are also used as an important marketing tool. Label designs are used to establish brand recognition and appeal to target groups. Product names and words such as "Light" and "Mild" mislead consumers about the health risks of smoking.

Two main provisions of the WHO FCTC focus on tobacco advertising and the use of misleading words on packaging. A few countries have already enacted comprehensive advertising bans, however, many others continue to allow the tobacco industry free rein.

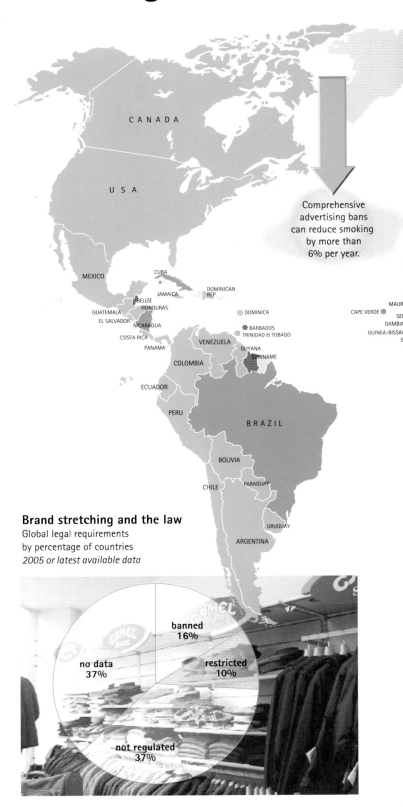

Comprehensive advertising bans can reduce smoking by more than 6% per year.

Brand stretching and the law
Global legal requirements by percentage of countries
2005 or latest available data

banned
16%

restricted
10%

no data
37%

not regulated
37%

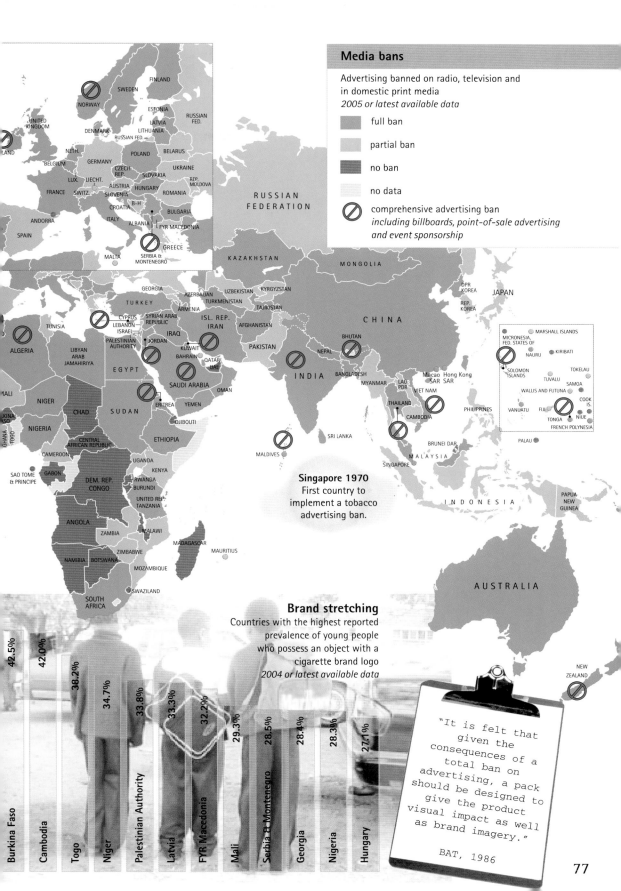

Media bans

Advertising banned on radio, television and in domestic print media
2005 or latest available data

- full ban
- partial ban
- no ban
- no data

comprehensive advertising ban
including billboards, point-of-sale advertising and event sponsorship

Singapore 1970
First country to implement a tobacco advertising ban.

Brand stretching
Countries with the highest reported prevalence of young people who possess an object with a cigarette brand logo
2004 or latest available data

Country	Percentage
Burkina Faso	42.5%
Cambodia	42.0%
Togo	38.2%
Niger	34.7%
Palestinian Authority	33.8%
Latvia	33.3%
FYR Macedonia	32.2%
Mali	29.3%
Serbia & Montenegro	28.5%
Georgia	28.4%
Nigeria	28.3%
Hungary	27.1%

"It is felt that given the consequences of a total ban on advertising, a pack should be designed to give the product visual impact as well as brand imagery."

BAT, 1986

"Plain packaging is important because it eliminates the positive imagery associated with the brand and potentially disrupts the process of smoking initiation whereby child smokers become brand loyal."
Rob Cunningham and Ken Kyle, 1995
Canadian Cancer Society

Since the 1960s, health warnings on cigarette packs have been used as a way to communicate risks associated with smoking. Warnings are now required in the majority of countries around the world and increasingly creative methods are being used to present these messages.

Cigarette packs in Brazil display graphic images, along with a phone number to a support centre for smokers wishing to quit. Australia's packs include cessation tips. The European Union is also encouraging member countries to use graphic health warnings, which have proven highly effective.

In order to be effective, warning labels should be regulated for size, content and design. Reports from Canada and Australia also suggest that plain packaging, displaying only the brand name and the health warning with no use of colour, logo, or graphic design, may increase both prominence and believability of health warnings. These health warnings should be extended to all forms of tobacco, including non-cigarette tobacco products.

In one of its strongest provisions, Article 11 of the WHO FCTC requires that tobacco product health warnings cover at least 30 percent, and preferably 50 percent, of the visible area on a cigarette pack. Misleading words implying a reduced health risk, such as "light" or "mild", are also banned.

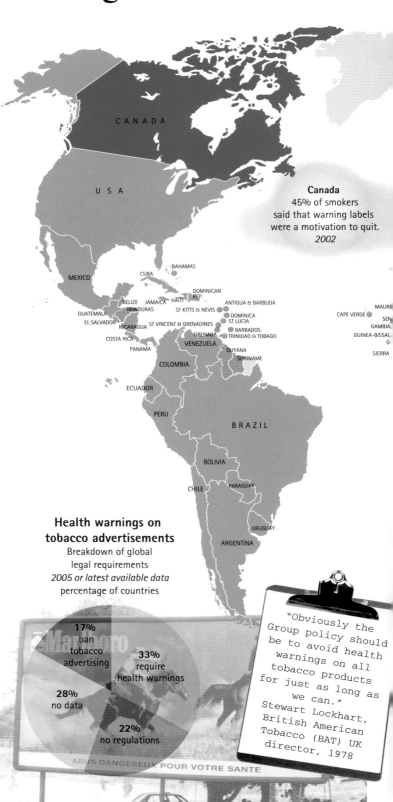

Canada
45% of smokers said that warning labels were a motivation to quit.
2002

Health warnings on tobacco advertisements
Breakdown of global legal requirements
2005 or latest available data
percentage of countries

17% ban tobacco advertising

33% require health warnings

28% no data

22% no regulations

"Obviously the Group policy should be to avoid health warnings on all tobacco products for just as long as we can."
Stewart Lockhart, British American Tobacco (BAT) UK director, 1978

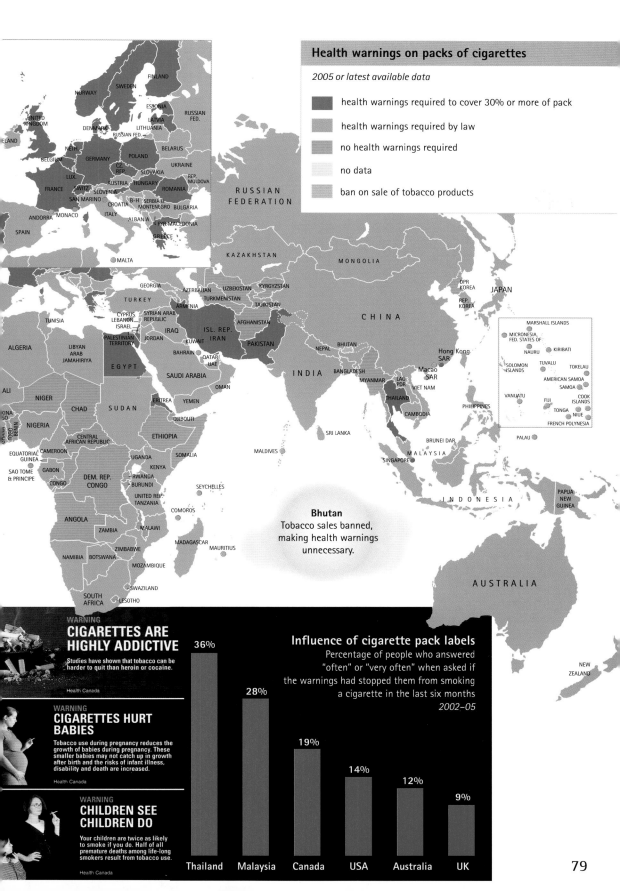

Health warnings on packs of cigarettes

2005 or latest available data

- health warnings required to cover 30% or more of pack
- health warnings required by law
- no health warnings required
- no data
- ban on sale of tobacco products

Bhutan
Tobacco sales banned, making health warnings unnecessary.

Map labels

FINLAND, SWEDEN, NORWAY, ESTONIA, RUSSIAN FED., LATVIA, LITHUANIA, UNITED KINGDOM, DENMARK, RUSSIAN FED., IRELAND, NETH., BELARUS, BELGIUM, GERMANY, POLAND, UKRAINE, LUX., CZ. REP., SLOVAKIA, FRANCE, SWITZ., AUSTRIA, HUNGARY, REP. MOLDOVA, SLOVENIA, ROMANIA, SAN MARINO, B-H, SERBIA &, CROATIA, MONTENEGRO, BULGARIA, ANDORRA, MONACO, ITALY, ALBANIA, SPAIN, FYR MACEDONIA, GREECE, MALTA

RUSSIAN FEDERATION, KAZAKHSTAN, MONGOLIA, GEORGIA, AZERBAIJAN, UZBEKISTAN, KYRGYZSTAN, DPR KOREA, JAPAN, TURKEY, ARMENIA, TURKMENISTAN, TAJIKISTAN, REP. KOREA, CYPRUS, SYRIAN ARAB REPUBLIC, AFGHANISTAN, CHINA, TUNISIA, LEBANON, ISRAEL, IRAQ, ISL. REP. IRAN, JORDAN, KUWAIT, PAKISTAN, NEPAL, BHUTAN, Hong Kong SAR, ALGERIA, LIBYAN ARAB JAMAHIRIYA, PALESTINIAN TERRITORY, BAHRAIN, QATAR, UAE, EGYPT, SAUDI ARABIA, INDIA, BANGLADESH, MYANMAR, LAO PDR, Macao SAR, VIET NAM, MALI, NIGER, OMAN, YEMEN, THAILAND, CHAD, SUDAN, ERITREA, PHILIPPINES, CAMBODIA, NIGERIA, DJIBOUTI, ETHIOPIA, SRI LANKA, BRUNEI DAR., CENTRAL AFRICAN REPUBLIC, SOMALIA, MALDIVES, MALAYSIA, EQUATORIAL GUINEA, CAMEROON, UGANDA, KENYA, SINGAPORE, SAO TOME & PRINCIPE, GABON, CONGO, RWANDA, BURUNDI, DEM. REP. CONGO, UNITED REP. TANZANIA, SEYCHELLES, INDONESIA, ANGOLA, COMOROS, PAPUA NEW GUINEA, ZAMBIA, MALAWI, MADAGASCAR, MAURITIUS, ZIMBABWE, NAMIBIA, BOTSWANA, MOZAMBIQUE, AUSTRALIA, SWAZILAND, SOUTH AFRICA, LESOTHO

MARSHALL ISLANDS, MICRONESIA, FED. STATES OF, KIRIBATI, NAURU, SOLOMON ISLANDS, TUVALU, TOKELAU, AMERICAN SAMOA, SAMOA, VANUATU, FIJI, COOK ISLANDS, TONGA, NIUE, FRENCH POLYNESIA, PALAU

NEW ZEALAND

Warnings (left column)

WARNING
CIGARETTES ARE HIGHLY ADDICTIVE
Studies have shown that tobacco can be harder to quit than heroin or cocaine.
Health Canada

WARNING
CIGARETTES HURT BABIES
Tobacco use during pregnancy reduces the growth of babies during pregnancy. These smaller babies may not catch up in growth after birth and the risks of infant illness, disability and death are increased.
Health Canada

WARNING
CHILDREN SEE CHILDREN DO
Your children are twice as likely to smoke if you do. Half of all premature deaths among life-long smokers result from tobacco use.
Health Canada

Influence of cigarette pack labels

Percentage of people who answered "often" or "very often" when asked if the warnings had stopped them from smoking a cigarette in the last six months
2002–05

Thailand	Malaysia	Canada	USA	Australia	UK
36%	28%	19%	14%	12%	9%

Education is essential for sustained progress in tobacco control. Legislative or tax interventions are unlikely to be effective if there is little public understanding of, and support for, such changes.

School programmes traditionally provide information about the harm caused by smoking, but this alone is not sufficient to change behaviour. A school tobacco control programme must prohibit tobacco use in school facilities and offer courses to build student confidence and social skills needed to resist cigarette marketing and peer pressure. Such courses should be part of a coordinated school health programme, reinforced by community-wide efforts.

Education is also important for teaching and understanding tobacco industry behaviour. Young people have the right to know that the tobacco industry designs youth marketing strategies to equate smoking with growing up, freedom, popularity, rebelliousness and being cool. To improve its public image, the tobacco industry recently introduced youth smoking-prevention programmes in more than half the countries in the world. These programmes portray smoking as acceptable adult behaviour, and suggest that young people should wait until they mature before deciding to smoke. Since young people aspire to be young adults, this type of message may actually encourage youth smoking.

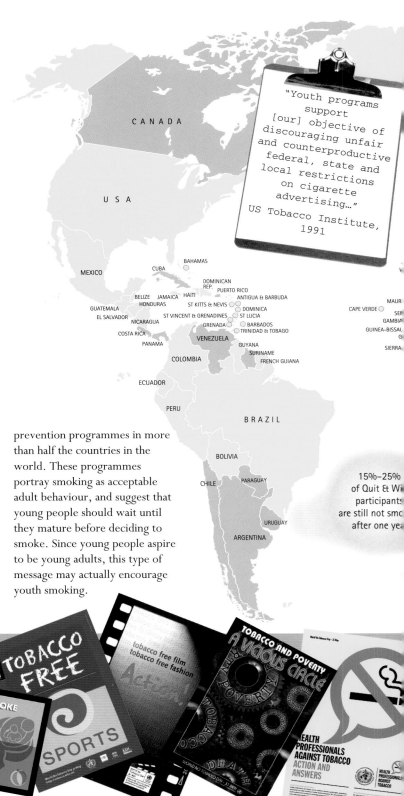

"Youth programs support [our] objective of discouraging unfair and counterproductive federal, state and local restrictions on cigarette advertising..."
US Tobacco Institute, 1991

15%–25% of Quit & Wi... participants... are still not smo... after one yea...

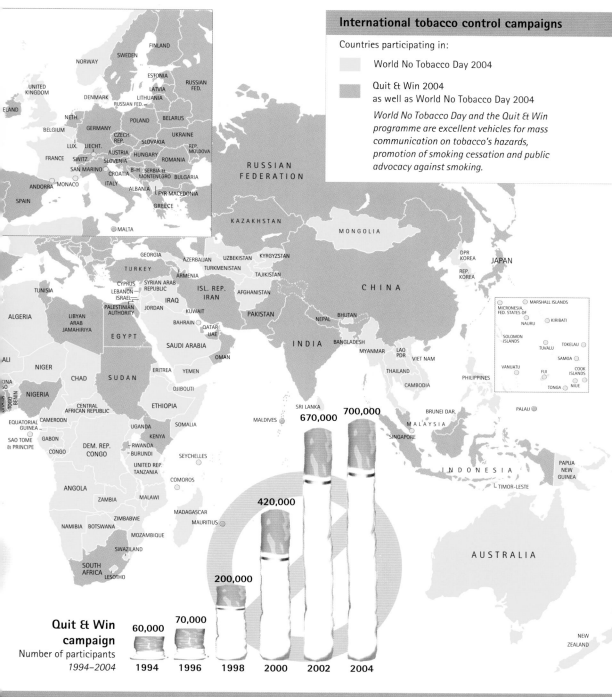

International tobacco control campaigns

Countries participating in:

World No Tobacco Day 2004

Quit & Win 2004
as well as World No Tobacco Day 2004

World No Tobacco Day and the Quit & Win programme are excellent vehicles for mass communication on tobacco's hazards, promotion of smoking cessation and public advocacy against smoking.

Quit & Win campaign
Number of participants
1994–2004

1994	1996	1998	2000	2002	2004
60,000	70,000	200,000	420,000	670,000	700,000

Annual themes of World No Tobacco Day: 31 May

1988 Tobacco or Health: Choose Health	**1995** The Economics of Tobacco	**2001** Secondhand Smoke Kills. Let's Clear the Air
1989 Women and Tobacco	**1996** Sports and the Arts Without Tobacco	**2002** Tobacco-Free Sports: Play it Clean
1990 Growing Up Without Tobacco		**2003** Tobacco-Free Film/ Tobacco-Free Fashion
1991 Tobacco in Public Places and on Public Transport	**1997** The United Nations and Specialized Agencies Against Tobacco "United for a Tobacco-Free World"	**2004** Tobacco and Poverty
1992 Tobacco at the Workplace	**1998** Growing Up Without Tobacco	**2005** Health Professionals in Tobacco Control
1993 Health Services, Including Health Personnel, Against Tobacco	**1999** Cessation	
1994 The Media Against Tobacco	**2000** The Entertainment Industry	

"Ill-health of body or of mind is defeat. Health alone is victory. Let all men, if they can manage it, contrive to be healthy!"
Thomas Carlyle, Scottish writer and journalist (1795–1881)

The main health hazards of smoking are reduced when smokers quit, even among those who have smoked for 30 or more years.

Smokers move through stages in relation to quitting: pre-contemplation, contemplation, readiness then action, followed by maintenance or relapse. Many move through this cycle several times before they finally quit successfully, while others report finding it easier to quit than they expected. These stages are influenced by increased costs due to tax increases, illness in the smoker, family or friends dying from tobacco, education through mass media, advice from health professionals, bans on promotion, creation of smoke-free areas and, while most smokers still quit on their own, availability of support and treatment.

There are now techniques to assist those who want to quit smoking, although these are not available in all parts of the world: social support, clinics, quitlines, internet sites; skills training; over-the-counter nicotine replacement therapy (NRT) and

prescription pharmaceutical treatments. While quitting smoking may be difficult for some, it certainly is possible. In some developed countries, there are actually more former smokers than current smokers.

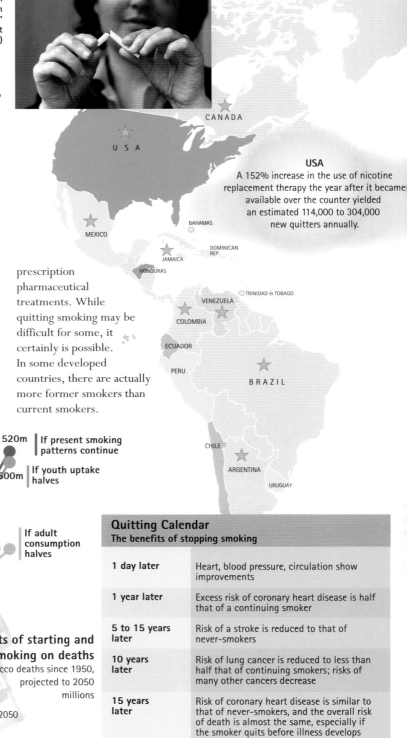

USA
A 152% increase in the use of nicotine replacement therapy the year after it became available over the counter yielded an estimated 114,000 to 304,000 new quitters annually.

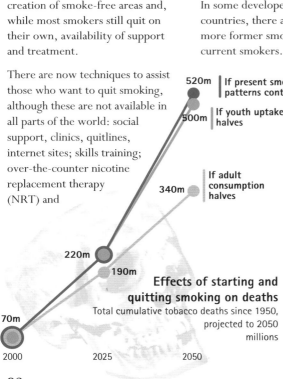

Effects of starting and quitting smoking on deaths
Total cumulative tobacco deaths since 1950, projected to 2050
millions

520m | If present smoking patterns continue
500m | If youth uptake halves
340m | If adult consumption halves
220m
190m
70m
2000 2025 2050

Quitting Calendar
The benefits of stopping smoking

1 day later	Heart, blood pressure, circulation show improvements
1 year later	Excess risk of coronary heart disease is half that of a continuing smoker
5 to 15 years later	Risk of a stroke is reduced to that of never-smokers
10 years later	Risk of lung cancer is reduced to less than half that of continuing smokers; risks of many other cancers decrease
15 years later	Risk of coronary heart disease is similar to that of never-smokers, and the overall risk of death is almost the same, especially if the smoker quits before illness develops

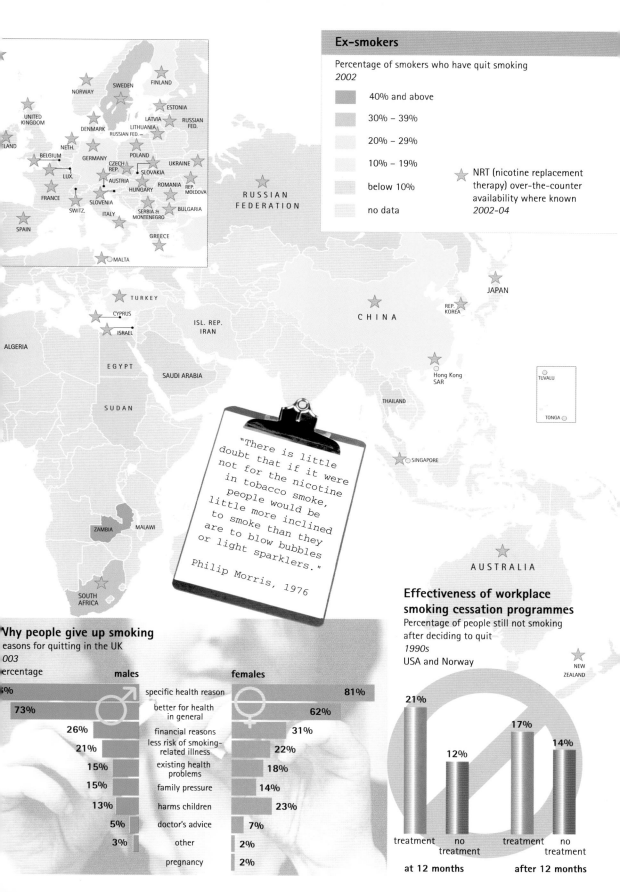

Ex-smokers

Percentage of smokers who have quit smoking
2002

- 40% and above
- 30% – 39%
- 20% – 29%
- 10% – 19%
- below 10%
- no data

⭐ NRT (nicotine replacement therapy) over-the-counter availability where known
2002–04

Map labels:

NORWAY, SWEDEN, FINLAND, ESTONIA, LATVIA, RUSSIAN FED., LITHUANIA, RUSSIAN FED., DENMARK, UNITED KINGDOM, ...ELAND, NETH., BELGIUM, LUX., GERMANY, POLAND, UKRAINE, CZECH REP., SLOVAKIA, AUSTRIA, ROMANIA, REP. MOLDOVA, HUNGARY, FRANCE, SWITZ., SLOVENIA, ITALY, SERBIA & MONTENEGRO, BULGARIA, SPAIN, GREECE, MALTA

RUSSIAN FEDERATION, TURKEY, CYPRUS, ISRAEL, ISL. REP. IRAN, ALGERIA, EGYPT, SAUDI ARABIA, SUDAN, ZAMBIA, MALAWI, SOUTH AFRICA

JAPAN, REP. KOREA, CHINA, Hong Kong SAR, THAILAND, TUVALU, TONGA, SINGAPORE, AUSTRALIA, NEW ZEALAND

> "There is little doubt that if it were not for the nicotine in tobacco smoke, people would be little more inclined to smoke than they are to blow bubbles or light sparklers."
>
> Philip Morris, 1976

Why people give up smoking

Reasons for quitting in the UK
2003
Percentage

	males	females
specific health reason	8%	81%
better for health in general	73%	62%
financial reasons	26%	31%
less risk of smoking-related illness	21%	22%
existing health problems	15%	18%
family pressure	15%	14%
harms children	13%	23%
doctor's advice	5%	7%
other	3%	2%
pregnancy		2%

Effectiveness of workplace smoking cessation programmes

Percentage of people still not smoking after deciding to quit
1990s
USA and Norway

at 12 months
- treatment: 21%
- no treatment: 12%

after 12 months
- treatment: 17%
- no treatment: 14%

Tobacco taxes

> "Sugar, rum and tobacco are commodities which are nowhere necessaries of life, which are become objects of almost universal consumption, and which are therefore extremely proper subjects of taxation."
> **Adam Smith** *An Inquiry into the Nature and Causes of the Wealth of Nations* 1776

P rice is the most important factor affecting short-term tobacco consumption patterns. A 10 percent increase in the price of cigarettes reduces consumption by about 4 percent in high-income countries and 8 percent in low and middle-income countries. Youth, minorities, and low-income smokers are two to three times more likely than other smokers to quit or smoke less in response to price increases. Because price is an especially powerful determinant of smoking initiation in youth, it significantly modulates long-term trends in cigarette consumption.

Higher tobacco taxes are easy to implement and usually generate higher tax receipts despite reducing cigarette consumption. This is good news for policy-makers seeking to protect public health but wary about losing an important source of government revenue.

The WHO's Framework Convention on Tobacco Control calls for ratifying states to adopt tax and price policies that reduce tobacco consumption. The World Bank proposes that taxes should account for two-thirds to four-fifths of the retail price of cigarettes. Although the tobacco industry claims that taxation leads to increased smuggling without dampening consumption, the evidence proves that, despite potential smuggling problems, tax increases significantly reduce cigarette consumption.

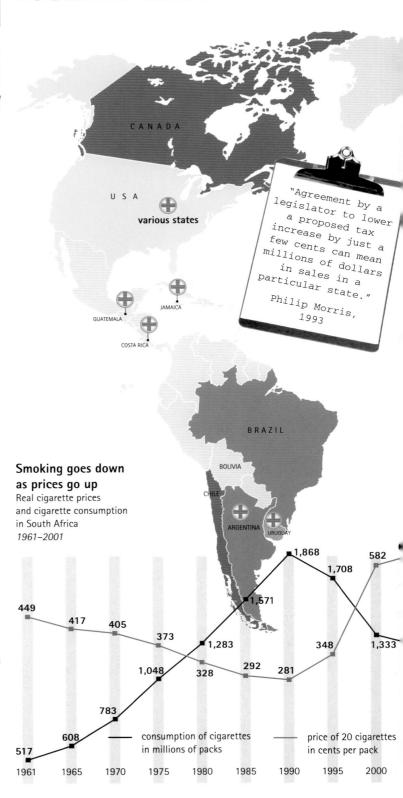

> "Agreement by a legislator to lower a proposed tax increase by just a few cents can mean millions of dollars in sales in a particular state."
> Philip Morris, 1993

Smoking goes down as prices go up
Real cigarette prices and cigarette consumption in South Africa
1961–2001

— consumption of cigarettes in millions of packs
— price of 20 cigarettes in cents per pack

Consumption: 517, 608, 783, 1,048, 1,283, 1,571, 1,868, 1,708, 1,333
Price: 449, 417, 405, 373, 328, 292, 281, 348, 582

1961 1965 1970 1975 1980 1985 1990 1995 2000

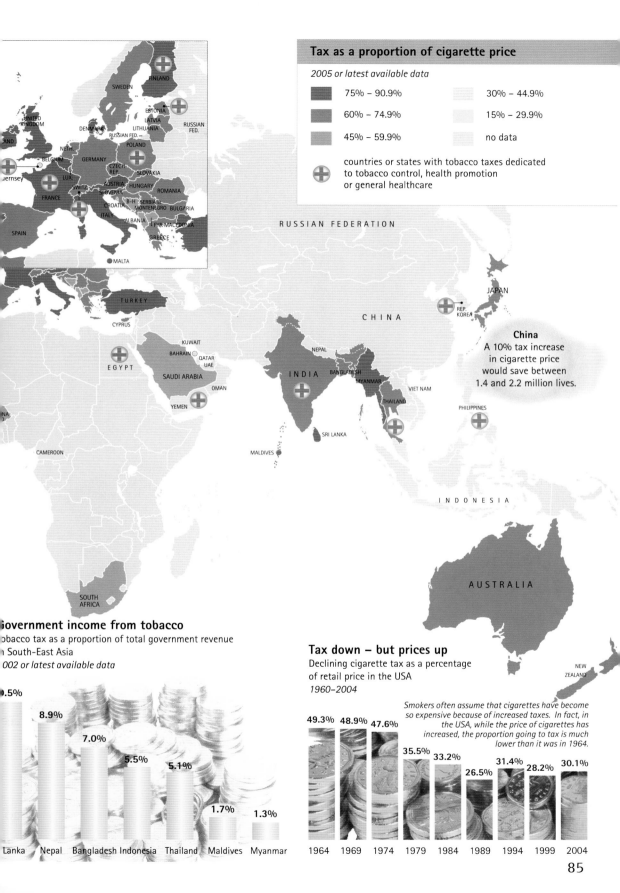

Tax as a proportion of cigarette price

2005 or latest available data

- 75% – 90.9%
- 60% – 74.9%
- 45% – 59.9%
- 30% – 44.9%
- 15% – 29.9%
- no data

⊕ countries or states with tobacco taxes dedicated to tobacco control, health promotion or general healthcare

Europe map labels

SWEDEN, FINLAND, UNITED KINGDOM, ESTONIA, LATVIA, LITHUANIA, RUSSIAN FED., RUSSIAN FED., DENMARK, NETH., BELGIUM, GERMANY, POLAND, Jersey, LUX., CZECH REP., SLOVAKIA, FRANCE, SWITZ., AUSTRIA, HUNGARY, ROMANIA, SLOVENIA, CROATIA, B-H, SERBIA & MONTENEGRO, BULGARIA, ITALY, ALBANIA, FYR-MACEDONIA, SPAIN, GREECE, MALTA

Main map labels

RUSSIAN FEDERATION, TURKEY, CYPRUS, KUWAIT, BAHRAIN, QATAR, UAE, EGYPT, SAUDI ARABIA, OMAN, YEMEN, NEPAL, CHINA, INDIA, BANGLADESH, MYANMAR, VIET NAM, THAILAND, SRI LANKA, MALDIVES, PHILIPPINES, JAPAN, REP. KOREA, CAMEROON, SOUTH AFRICA, INDONESIA, AUSTRALIA, NEW ZEALAND

China
A 10% tax increase in cigarette price would save between 1.4 and 2.2 million lives.

Government income from tobacco

Tobacco tax as a proportion of total government revenue in South-East Asia
2002 or latest available data

- ...5% — Sri Lanka
- 8.9% — Nepal
- 7.0% — Bangladesh
- 5.5% — Indonesia
- 5.1% — Thailand
- 1.7% — Maldives
- 1.3% — Myanmar

Tax down – but prices up

Declining cigarette tax as a percentage of retail price in the USA
1960–2004

Smokers often assume that cigarettes have become so expensive because of increased taxes. In fact, in the USA, while the price of cigarettes has increased, the proportion going to tax is much lower than it was in 1964.

Year	Percentage
1964	49.3%
1969	48.9%
1974	47.6%
1979	35.5%
1984	33.2%
1989	26.5%
1994	31.4%
1999	28.2%
2004	30.1%

"Tobacco litigation enables the citizens of each country to learn about misbehaviour by the international tobacco cartel that was directed specifically at them."
Professor Richard Daynard, Northeastern University, USA, 2005

The modern era of tobacco litigation began with a personal injury lawsuit in the USA in 1954. For more than 40 years the tobacco industry boasted it had not lost a single case, but a seminal judgement in a Minnesota case that began in 1994 released millions of pages of internal tobacco industry documents into the public domain. These documents revealed that tobacco companies actively concealed their knowledge about the harmfulness of smoking and deceived governments, the media and their clients – smokers – about the extent of death and disease caused by their products.

Litigation has put the industry on the defensive, forced tobacco companies to the bargaining table, and resulted in the industry paying US states billions of dollars per year. In 1999, the US government filed a landmark lawsuit against the major cigarette companies to hold them accountable for a half century of illegal and harmful practices, including conspiracy to conceal the health risks and addictiveness of their products, defrauding smokers, and marketing cigarettes to children. The decision is still pending.

Although still a new phenomenon in countries other than the USA, tobacco litigation is clearly increasing around the world. For example, Australia has seen major rulings on passive smoking and public interest litigation is rising in France, India, Niger and Uganda.

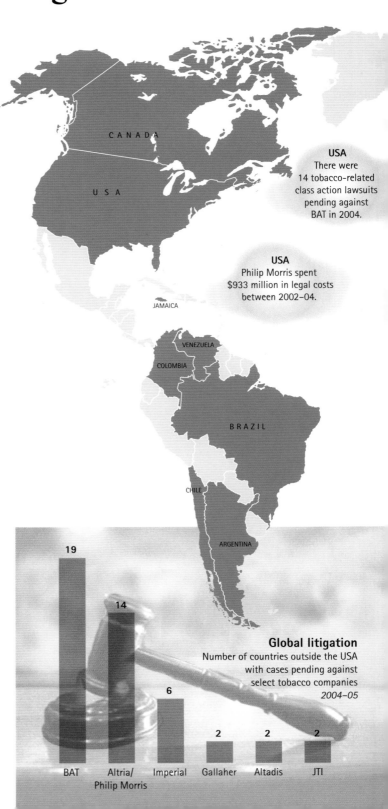

USA
There were 14 tobacco-related class action lawsuits pending against BAT in 2004.

USA
Philip Morris spent $933 million in legal costs between 2002–04.

Global litigation
Number of countries outside the USA with cases pending against select tobacco companies
2004–05

BAT	19
Altria/Philip Morris	14
Imperial	6
Gallaher	2
Altadis	2
JTI	2

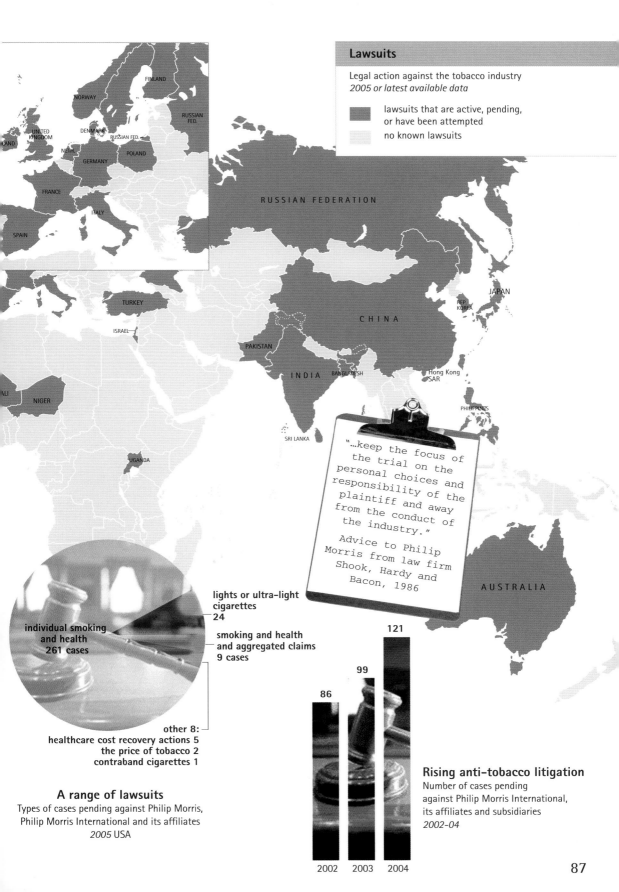

lawsuits that are active, pending, or have been attempted

no known lawsuits

FINLAND

NORWAY

RUSSIAN FED.

UNITED KINGDOM

DENMARK

RUSSIAN FED.

NETH.

GERMANY

POLAND

FRANCE

ITALY

SPAIN

RUSSIAN FEDERATION

TURKEY

JAPAN

ISRAEL

REP. KOREA

CHINA

PAKISTAN

INDIA   BANGLADESH

Hong Kong SAR

MALI

NIGER

SRI LANKA

PHILIPPINES

UGANDA

AUSTRALIA

"...keep the focus of the trial on the personal choices and responsibility of the plaintiff and away from the conduct of the industry."

Advice to Philip Morris from law firm Shook, Hardy and Bacon, 1986

lights or ultra-light cigarettes
24

individual smoking and health
261 cases

smoking and health and aggregated claims
9 cases

other 8:
healthcare cost recovery actions 5
the price of tobacco 2
contraband cigarettes 1

A range of lawsuits
Types of cases pending against Philip Morris, Philip Morris International and its affiliates
2005 USA

121

99

86

2002   2003   2004

Rising anti-tobacco litigation
Number of cases pending against Philip Morris International, its affiliates and subsidiaries
2002-04

"There will be 1 billion deaths from tobacco in the 21st century unless strong and sustained action is taken now."
Richard Peto and Alan Lopez, 2002

Future predictions are by their nature speculative, but some things are certain: the epidemic, with its attendant health and economic burden, is both increasing and also shifting from developed to developing nations; and more women are smoking.

The industry is consolidating, and also shifting from the west to developing regions, where there may be less government control and public debate about the role of transnational tobacco companies.

The future looks bleak; the global tobacco epidemic is worse today than it was 50 years ago. And it will be even worse in another 50 years unless an extraordinary effort is made now. The number of smokers in the world will inexorably rise, principally because of population expansion.

Many countries, including developing countries, have already shown that smoking rates can be reduced. These successes can be reproduced by any responsible nation, but only through immediate, determined, and sustained governmental and community action. The future is uncertain and some of the events predicted here may never occur, but there must be the political will to tackle tobacco, and appropriate funding proportional to the magnitude of the epidemic, as well as individual commitment by smokers to quit. In the words of Norway's seasoned advocate Dr Kjell Bjartveit, "It can be done."

	2000–2010	2010–2020
Number of smokers		Deaths from tobacco use are predicted to double between 2005 and 2020, from 5 million to 10 million a year.
— assuming constant prevalence and medium variant projected population		1.6b
— assuming reduced prevalence of 1% per year, medium variant projected population	1.4b / 1.3b	1.4b
Health	Tobacco causes 5 million deaths annually. Tobacco causes 8.8% of all global deaths and 4.2% of disability. More than 700 million children exposed to passive smoking at home.	Individuals genetically prone to tobacco-related diseases can be identified at birth. Previously untreatable cancers can now be treated. New technologies for diagnosis and treatment are expensive and have little impact on global mortality trends.
Economics	Global economic costs of tobacco: US$500 billion a year by 2010.	Tobacco-related illnesses rise to top health expenditure in many countries. Many governments conclude the economic of tobacco outweigh any benefit. A severe economic depression and/or a ma international security crisis cause attention tobacco control issues to temporarily dimi
Tobacco industry	Attempts to produce genetically modified tobacco. Some tobacco companies buy pharmaceutical companies. The industry tries to re-position its public image as changed and socially responsible. Some tobacco companies seek regulation on their own terms.	Industry consolidation leads to two or thre huge conglomerates accounting for the bulk of global sales. Continued privatisation sees end of state-run tobacco companies. Niche markets still exist for smaller player (e.g. cigars, snus). Liberalization of global trade rules welcomed by the industry. Smuggled cigarettes overtake legal sales.
Action taken	The WHO Framework Convention on Tobacco Control ratified by most countries. Most countries ban smoking in all public places and workplaces. Incentives for quitting include monetary savings through rebates and lower health insurance premiums. In many countries, there is a gradual shift in the perception of smoking as it is no longer the norm.	Tobacco advertising and promotion are eliminated worldwide. Vaccine produced to switch off nicotine receptors. Medical schools globally introduce systematic teaching on tobacco. Smoke-free areas become the norm. Cigarette packets will be plain black and white and contain only brand name and explicit health warnings. Tobacco-dependent economies are assisted in diversifying. Nicotine Replacement Therapy sold over the counter worldwide.

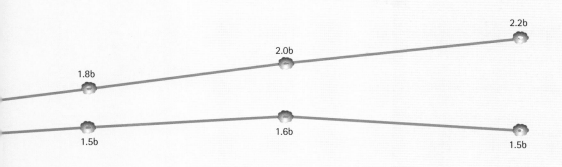

1.8b

2.0b

2.2b

1.5b

1.6b

1.5b

Tobacco causes 10 million deaths annually.

Spectacular advances are made in the investigation, diagnosis and treatment of tobacco-related diseases e.g. genetics, surgery, nanotechnology, telemedicine, targeted pharmaceuticals and radiotherapy, but these advances have minimal effect on global tobacco-related mortality.

New global virus pandemic temporarily pushes tobacco issues completely off the public health agenda.

770 million children exposed to passive smoking at home.

Number of cumulative deaths from tobacco:

• if present trends continue: 520 million
• if proportion of young adults taking up smoking halves by 2020: 500 million
• if adult consumption halves by 2020: 340 million

The gap between rich and poor countries grows as health services in poor countries collapse under the strain of tobacco disease and deaths.

Governments realize destructive effects of tobacco on national economies.

Global economic costs of tobacco: US$1 trillion a year.

Healthcare costs for treating tobacco-related diseases among smokers and former smokers surpass all other healthcare expenditures.

Much of the developed world moves to a managed tobacco industry, with tobacco-attributable healthcare costs reimbursed and compensation paid to individual smokers and non-smokers harmed by tobacco.

Cigarettes only available on prescription in rich countries.

The tobacco industry is fully regulated, with licensing of nicotine as an addictive drug, and manufacture, promotion and sale under strict regulatory control by government agencies.

Huge advances are made in genetics. The tobacco plant becomes key to producing vaccines and other beneficial medical products.

World's top tobacco companies now based in Asia.

Almost no tobacco is grown in the USA.

New, commercially profitable uses for tobacco are found that do not harm human health.

Tobacco control funded from a percentage of tobacco tax in many countries.

"Duty Free" tobacco no longer exists.

Health education messages are more skilful, hard-hitting, and disseminated more effectively.

In every country, the tax on tobacco is at least 75% of the retail price.

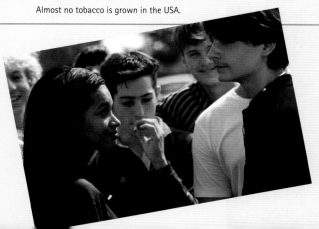

6000 BCE *Americas* First cultivation of the tobacco plant.

circa 1 BCE *Americas* Indigenous Americans began smoking and using tobacco enemas.

Americas Huron Indian myth: "In ancient times, when the land was barren and the people were starving, the Great Spirit sent forth a woman to save humanity. As she travelled over the world everywhere her right hand touched the soil, there grew potatoes. And everywhere her left hand touched the soil, there grew corn. And in the place where she had sat, there grew tobacco."

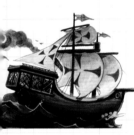

1492 Christopher Columbus and his crew returned to Europe from the Americas with the first tobacco leaves and seeds ever seen on the continent. A crew member, Rodrigo de Jerez, was seen smoking and imprisoned by the Inquisition, which believed he was possessed by the devil.

Early 1500s: *Middle East* Tobacco introduced when the Turks took it to Egypt.

1530-1600 *China* Tobacco introduced via Japan or the Philippines.

1558 *Europe* Tobacco plant brought to Europe. Attempts at cultivation failed.

1560 *Africa* Portuguese and Spanish traders introduced tobacco to Africa.

1560 *France* Diplomat Jean Nicot, Lord of Villemain, introduced tobacco from Portugal. Queen Catherine de Medici used it to treat her migraines.

1577 *Europe* European doctors recommended tobacco as a cure for toothache, falling fingernails, worms, halitosis, lockjaw and cancer.

1592–1598 *Korea* The Japanese Army introduced tobacco into Korea.

circa 1600 *India* Tobacco first introduced.

1603 *Japan* Use of tobacco well-established.

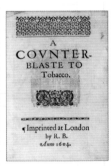

1604 *England* King James I wrote *A Counterblaste to Tobacco*. "Smoking is a custom loathsome to the eye, hateful to the nose, harmful to the brain, dangerous to the lungs, and in the black, stinking fume thereof nearest resembling the horrible Stygian smoke of the pit that is bottomless."

1600s *China* Philosopher Fang Yizhi pointed out that long years of smoking "scorches one's lung."

1608–1609 *Japan* Ban on smoking introduced to prevent fires.

1612 *Americas* Tobacco first grown commercially.

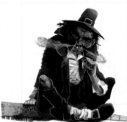

1614 *England* 7,000 tobacco shops opened with the first sale of Virginia tobacco.

1633 *Turkey* Death penalty imposed for smoking.

1634 *China* Qing Dynasty decreed a smoking ban during which a violator was executed. This was not to protect health, but to address the inequality of trade with Korea.

1650s *South Africa* European settlers grew tobacco and used it as a form of currency.

1692 and 1717 *Korea* Bans on smoking in Choson introduced to reduce fire risk.

circa 1710 *Russia* Peter the Great encouraged his courtiers to smoke tobacco and drink coffee, which was seen as fashionable and pro-European.

1700s *Africa/Americas* African slaves forced to work in tobacco fields.

1719 *France* Smoking was prohibited in many places.

1753 *Sweden* Botanist Carolus Linnaeus named the plant genus nicotiana and describes two species, nicotiana rustica and nicotiana tabacum.

1761 *England* First study of the effects of tobacco by Dr John Hill; snuff users were warned they risked nasal cancers.

1769 *New Zealand* Captain James Cook arrived smoking a pipe, and was promptly doused in case he was a demon.

1771 *France* French official was condemned to be hanged for admitting foreign tobacco into the country.

1788 *Australia* Tobacco arrived with the First Fleet, eleven ships which sailed from England carrying mostly convicts and crew.

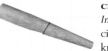

1795 Sammuel Thomas von Soemmering reported cancers of the lip in pipe smokers.

18th century Snuff was the most popular mode of tobacco use.

1800 *Canada* Tobacco first grown commercially.

1833 *UK* Phosphorus friction matches introduced on a commercial scale, making smoking more convenient.

1840 *France* Frederic Chopin's mistress, the Baroness de Dudevant, likely to have been the first woman to smoke in public (in Paris).

1847 *England* Philip Morris Esq, a tobacconist and importer of fine cigars, opened a shop in London selling hand-rolled Turkish cigarettes.

1854 *England* Philip Morris began making his own cigarettes. Old Bond Street soon became the centre of the retail tobacco trade.

1858 *China* Treaty of Tianjin allowed cigarettes to be imported into China duty-free.

1862 *USA* First federal tobacco tax was introduced to help finance the Civil War.

1876 *Korea* Foreign cigarettes and matches were introduced.

1880s *England* Richard Benson and William Hedges opened a tobacconist shop near Philip Morris in London.

1881 *USA* First practical cigarette-making machine patented by James Bonsack. It could produce 120,000 cigarettes a day, each machine doing the work of 48 people. Production costs plummeted, and – with the invention of the safety match a few decades later – cigarette-smoking began its explosive growth.

circa 1890s *Indonesia* Clove cigarette, the kretek, invented.

before 1900 Lung cancer was extremely rare.

1901–02 *England* Imperial Tobacco Company Limited (ITL) and British American Tobacco (BAT) were founded.

1903 *Brazil* Tobacco company Souza Cruz founded.

1913 *USA* Birth of the "modern" cigarette: RJ Reynolds introduced the Camel brand.

1915 *Japan* Cancer was induced in laboratory animals for the first time by applying coal tar to rabbits' skin at Tokyo University.

1921 *Korea* Korea Ginseng Corporation became Korea Tobacco and Ginseng (KTG) and a monopoly was formed.

1924 Philip Morris introduced Marlboro as a women's cigarette as "mild as May."

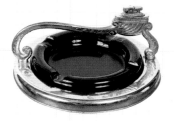

1924 Reader's Digest published *Does Tobacco Injure the Human Body*, the beginning of a Reader's Digest campaign to make people think before starting to smoke.

1929 *USA* Edward Bernays mounted a "freedom march" of smoking debutantes/fashion models who walk down Fifth Avenue in New York during the Easter parade dressed as Statues of Liberty and holding aloft their Lucky Strike cigarettes as "torches of freedom."

1929 *Germany* Fritz Lickint of Dresden published the first formal statistical evidence of a lung cancer–tobacco link, based on a case series showing that lung-cancer sufferers were likely to be smokers.

1936 *Germany* Fritz Lickint first used the term "Passivrauchen" (passive smoking) in *Tabakgenuß und Gesundheit*.

1939 *USA* Tobacco companies found price-fixing.

1939 *USA* Drs Alton Ochsner and Michael DeBakey first reported the association of smoking and lung cancer.

1947 *Canada* Dr Norman Delarue compared 50 patients with lung cancer with 50 patients hospitalized with other diseases. He discovered that over 90% of the first group – but only half of the second – were smokers, and confidently predicted that by 1950 no one would be smoking.

1950–1994

1950 *USA* The link between smoking and lung cancer was confirmed. A landmark article "Tobacco smoking as a possible etiologic factor in bronchogenic carcinoma" by E L Wynder and Evarts Graham was published in *The Journal of the American Medical Association*. The same issue featured a full-page ad for Chesterfields with the actress Gene Tierney and golfer Ben Hogan; the journal accepted tobacco ads until 1953.

1951 *UK* Dr Richard Doll and Prof Austin Bradford Hill conducted the first large-scale case control study on the link between smoking and lung cancer.

1953 *USA* Tobacco executives met in New York City to find a way to deal with recent scientific data pointing to the health hazards of cigarettes.

1950s *China* State monopoly takes control of the tobacco business, and foreign tobacco companies left China. BAT, almost half of whose revenues came from China, was especially hurt.

1954 *USA* St Louis factory worker Ira C Lowe filed the first product liability action against a tobacco company on behalf of her smoker husband who died from cancer. The tobacco company won.

1954 *USA* The Marlboro cowboy was created for Philip Morris by Chicago ad agency Leo Burnett.

1954 *USA* Tobacco Industry Research Committee (TIRC) placed a nationwide two-page ad:

"A frank statement to cigarette smokers."

1957 *Vatican* Pope Pius XII suggested that the Jesuit order give up smoking.

1958 *USA* Tobacco Institute formed.

1960 *USA* Framingham Heart Study found cigarette smoking increased the risk of heart disease.

1962 *UK* First Report of the Royal College of Physicians of London on Smoking and Health.

1963 *World Tobacco* and *Tobacco Journal International*, tobacco industry trade journals, first published.

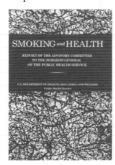

1964 *USA* First US Surgeon General's report on smoking and health announced that smoking caused lung cancer in men.

1965 WHO established the International Agency for Research on Cancer (IARC) based in Lyons, France.

1965 *UK* Cigarette advertising on TV was banned.

1967 *USA (New York)* First World Conference on Tobacco or Health.

1969 *USA* Surgeon General's Report confirmed the link between maternal smoking and low birth weight.

1971 *UK* ASH UK established, the first national tobacco control organization.

1971 *USA* Cigarette manufacturers first agreed to put health warning

on advertisements. This agreement was later made law.

1972 Marlboro became the best-selling cigarette in the world.

1972 International Association for the Study of Lung Cancer was inaugurated.

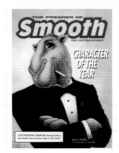

1974 *France* Joe Camel was born – used in French poster campaign for Camel cigarettes.

1976 *USA* Shimp v New Jersey Bell Telephone Co filed, the world's first lawsuit regarding second-hand smoke. The office worker was granted an injunction to ensure a smoke-free area in her workplace.

1977 *Italy* The Martignacco Project community prevention trial resulted in a reduction of coronary heart disease.

1977 *USA* First Great American Smokeout held nationally, during which smokers quit smoking on the third Thursday of November.

1978 *Australia* The three-year community study North Coast Healthy Lifestyle Programme showed a significant reduction in smoking.

1978 *USA* A Roper Report prepared for the Tobacco Institute concluded that the non-smokers' rights movement was "the most dangerous development to the viability of the tobacco industry that has yet occurred."

1979 *USA* Tobacco Control Resource Center and its Tobacco Products Liability Project was formed.

1979 The Freedom Organization for the Right to Enjoy Smoking Tobacco (FOREST) formed.

1979 *Australia* Activist group BUGAUP (Billboard Utilising Graffitists Against Unhealthy Promotions) was formed, re-facing tobacco and alcohol billboards.

1981 *Japan* Professor Takeshi Hirayama (1923–1995) published

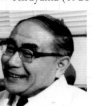

the first report linking passive smoking and lung cancer in the non-smoking wives of men who smoked.

1983 *Europe* ERC Group plc, an independent market research group, published first European Tobacco Market Report.

1984 Nicotine gum was first introduced.

1985 *USA* Lung cancer surpassed breast cancer as number one cancer killer of women.

by 1985 73% of the world's tobacco was grown in developing countries.

1987 *USA* Smoke-free Educational Services founded, advocating the right of all employees to work in a safe, healthy, smoke-free environment.

1988 First WHO report on the effects of smokeless tobacco.

1988 *USA* Framingham Heart Study found cigarette smoking increased the risk of stroke.

1988 First WHO World No Tobacco Day, subsequently an annual event on 31 May, with different annual themes and awards of commemorative medals.

1989 *Asia* The Asia Pacific Association for the Control of

Tobacco (APACT) was established by Dr David Yen of the John Tung Foundation, Taiwan, China.

1990 GLOBALink inaugurated, the international interactive website and marketplace founded by the International Union Against Cancer for the international tobacco-control community.

1990 International Network of Women Against Tobacco (INWAT) formed.

1990 *China* Chinese Association on Smoking and Health inaugurated.

1991 *UK* International Agency on Tobacco and Health (IATH) formed to act as an information and advisory service for the least developed countries.

1991 Realization that chemicals in cigarette smoke switch on a gene that makes lung cells vulnerable to the chemicals' cancer-causing properties.

1991 International Network towards Smoke-free Hospitals inaugurated, aiming to give healthy environment to hospital staff and patients.

1992 *Tobacco Control* journal founded by the British Medical Journals group. This was the first international peer-reviewed journal on tobacco control, and in 2004, the journal had the highest impact factor of all in the substance abuse field.

1992 *Northern Ireland*, *UK* First conference on women and tobacco initiated by the UICC (International Union Against Cancer), the Ulster Cancer

Foundation and the Health Promotion Agency of Northern Ireland.

1993 *USA* Environmental Protection Agency (EPA) declared cigarette smoke a Class-A carcinogen.

1993 *South Africa* Tobacco Products Control Amendment Act passed.

1993 *Europe* European Network on Young People and Tobacco (ENYPAT) founded.

1994 *USA* Cigarette executives testified before Congress that in their opinion nicotine was not addictive.

1994 Society for Research on Nicotine and Tobacco founded.

1994 *USA* Confidential internal tobacco industry documents leaked to Professor Stan Glantz.

1994 *Austria* First TABEXPO held in Vienna. TABEXPO stages exhibitions and congresses for the international tobacco industry.

1994 International Non Governmental Coalition Against Tobacco (INGCAT) founded.

1994 First international "Quit &Win" campaign.

1994 *Canada* Research for International Tobacco Control (RITC) inaugurated, with a major focus on developing countries.

1994 *USA* State of Mississippi filed first lawsuit by a health authority for reimbursement of money expended to treat smokers with smoking-caused illnesses. It ended with an out-of-court settlement.

1995–2006

1995 *USA* Smokescreen.org (later Smoke-free.net) was inaugurated. Focusing on the right to breathe clean air, this was the first web-based advocacy site that enabled visitors to send faxes directly to their elected officials. Mainly used by Americans, but also by 10,000 international participants.

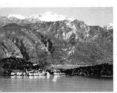

1995 *Italy* The Bellagio statement on tobacco and sustainable development was issued by members of retreat at Rockefeller Foundation's Bellagio Study and Conference Centre.

1995 International Council of Nurses (ICN) published position statement on tobacco.

1995 *USA* Federal Drug Administration declared cigarettes to be "drug delivery devices." Restrictions were proposed on marketing and sales to reduce smoking by young people.

1990s Cigars became fashionable again.

1995 Forces International (Fight Ordinances and Restrictions to Control and Eliminate Smoking), an ostensibly grassroots pro-tobacco organization unaffiliated with the tobacco industry, established.

1995 *USA* "Marlboro Man" David McLean died of lung cancer.

1996 *USA* First smoking cessation guideline, issued by the Public Health Service, Federal Government.

1997 *Europe* European Network for Smoking Prevention (ENSP) created.

1997 *UK (Scotland)* Doctors and Tobacco: Tobacco Control Resource Centre (TCRC) formed by the European Forum Medical Associations (EFMA). The TCRC is based at the British Medical Association in Edinburgh, and works in partnership with national medical associations across Europe.

1997 *USA* Congress passed a bill prohibiting the Departments of State, Justice and Commerce from promoting the sale or export of tobacco.

1998 Studies confirmed the harmfulness of smoking fewer than 10 cigarettes a day.

1998 WHO's Tobacco-free Initiative (TFI) was established.

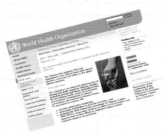

1998 United Nations Foundation first funded a tobacco control project.

1998 *Australia* Tobacco Control Supersite website inaugurated, enabling exploration of internal, previously private tobacco industry documents, and providing access to a wide range of information relevant to smoking prevention and control in Australia.

1998 *USA* Master Settlement Agreement between Attorneys General of 46 states and five territories with tobacco companies to settle lawsuits.

1999 *USA* Network for Accountability of Tobacco Transnationals (NATT) founded by Infact, made up of environmental, consumers, human rights and corporate accountability organizations working together to forge new ground in international law to prevent life-threatening abuses by transnational corporations.

1999 Global Youth Tobacco Surveys (GYTS) commenced.

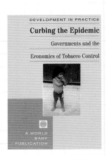

1999 World Bank report: *Curbing the Epidemic: Governments and the Economics of Tobacco Control.*

1999 *Sweden* Swedish International Development Cooperation Agency (Sida) first supported tobacco control projects.

1999 *UK* Britain's royal family ordered the removal of its seal of approval and royal crest from Gallaher's Benson and Hedges cigarettes by 2000.

1999 *USA* US Justice Department sued the tobacco industry to recover billions of government dollars spent on smoking-related healthcare, accusing cigarette-makers of a "coordinated campaign of fraud and deceit."

2000 Framework Convention Alliance (FCA) of NGOs formed to support the WHO Framework Convention on Tobacco Control (FCTC) and related protocols.

2000 *USA* First Luther L Terry Awards for contributions to tobacco control.

2000 Global Partnerships for Tobacco Control founded by Essential Action to help support and strengthen international tobacco control activities at the grass roots level.

2000 International Tobacco Evidence Network (ITEN) established, with the goal of expanding global research.

2000 Rockefeller Foundation International Health Research Awards for "Trading Tobacco for Health" in selected ASEAN countries.

2000 *South Africa* Tobacco Products Control Amendment Act came into effect, strictly regulating smoking and advertising.

2001 South-East Asia Tobacco Control Alliance (SEATCA) formed to act as supportive base for government and non-government tobacco control workers and advocates.

2001 *USA* Clearing the Smoke: Assessing the Science Base for Tobacco Harm Reduction, a new report from the Institute of Medicine (IOM) was released.

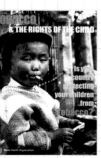

2001 WHO published *Tobacco & the Rights of the Child*.

2001 *Czech Republic* Philip Morris released a report to the government that concluded that smokers save the state money – by dying early.

2002 TobaccoPedia, the online tobacco encyclopaedia, was inaugurated.

2002 *USA* Global Tobacco Research Network founded by the Institute for Global Tobacco Control at Johns Hopkins University.

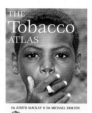

2002 WHO published the first edition of *The Tobacco Atlas*.

2002 *USA* Fogarty International Centre, National Institutes of Health, allocated funding for tobacco research projects.

2003 World Medical Association launched "The Doctors' Manifesto for Global Tobacco Control."

2003 Treatobacco web-based database and educational resource for treatment of tobacco dependence established by the Society for Research on Nicotine and Tobacco.

2003 The Global Network of Pharmacists Against Tobacco launched.

2004 *Ireland* Workplace smoking ban, including pubs and restaurants, implemented. Exactly one year after the ban, cigarette sales had declined by 18%.

2004 First general textbook for health professionals on tobacco published: *Tobacco: Science, Policy and Public Health*.

2004 *Europe* The EU Commission published the ASPECT report, *Tobacco or Health in the European Union: Past, Present and Future,* the first comprehensive overview of tobacco control in the 25 EU member countries plus Norway, Iceland and Switzerland.

2004 *Uganda* Environment Minister Kahinda Otafiire announced a ban on smoking in restaurants, educational institutions and bars.

2004 *Canada* Non-Smokers' Rights Association, founded in 1974, the first such association, celebrated its 30th anniversary.

2004 Myriad Editions created interactive internet mapping of *The Tobacco Atlas* launched by Global Tobacco Research Network, Johns Hopkins University.

2004 WHO's "Code of practice on tobacco control for health professional organizations" launched.

2004 IARC Monograph on Tobacco Smoke and Involuntary Smoking released, conclusively refuting extensive tobacco industry disinformation.

2004 *India* Complete ban on tobacco advertising and promotions came into effect.

2005 World Dental Federation (FDI) launches Tobacco or Oral Health publication.

2005 WHO Framework Convention on Tobacco Control 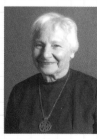 (FCTC) came into force, using international law to reduce tobacco use. This convention was initiated by Ruth Roemer in 1993.

2006 Second edition of *The Tobacco Atlas* published by American Cancer Society in print and online at www.tobaccoresearch.net/atlas

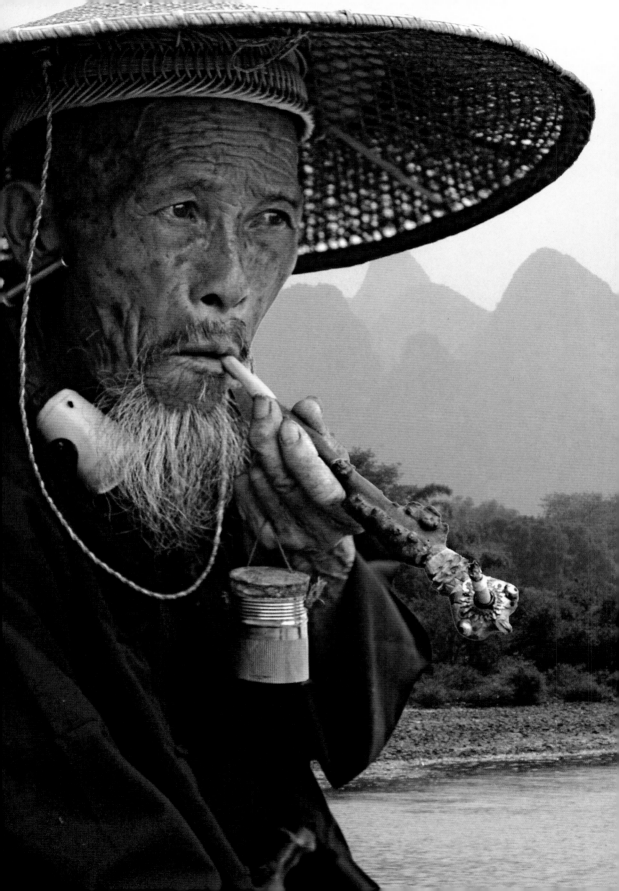

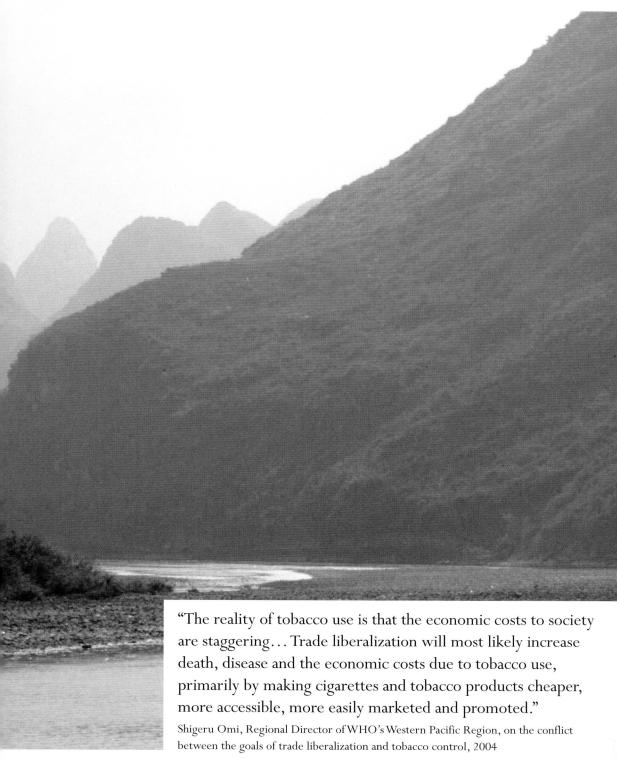

PART SIX

WORLD TABLES

"The reality of tobacco use is that the economic costs to society are staggering… Trade liberalization will most likely increase death, disease and the economic costs due to tobacco use, primarily by making cigarettes and tobacco products cheaper, more accessible, more easily marketed and promoted."

Shigeru Omi, Regional Director of WHO's Western Pacific Region, on the conflict between the goals of trade liberalization and tobacco control, 2004

Table A The demographics of tobacco

Countries	1 Population thousands	2 Adult smoking prevalence percentages			Age span years	3 Health professionals' smoking prevalence percentages
		total	male	female		
Afghanistan	20,988	49.5%	82.0%	17.0%	–	–
Albania	3,169	39.0%	60.0%	18.0%	15+	43.3%
Algeria	31,833	12.8%	32.3%	0.4%	25–64	37.0%
Angola	13,522	–	–	–	–	–
Antigua and Barbuda	79	–	–	–	–	–
Argentina	36,772	28.5%	32.3%	24.9%	18–64	30.3%
Armenia	3,056	32.1%	61.8%	2.4%	18+	56.8%
Australia	19,881	17.4%	18.6%	16.3%	18+	3.2%
Austria	8,090	29.1%	33.9%	24.2%	25–64	10.7%
Azerbaijan	8,233	–	–	0.6%	–	–
Bahrain	712	10.2%	15.0%	3.1%	15+	14.6%
Bangladesh	138,066	40.8%	54.8%	26.7%	18+	22.2%
Barbados	271	8.5%	20.1%	0.8%	25+	–
Belarus	9,881	27.3%	53.2%	7.1%	–	–
Belgium	10,376	27.0%	30.0%	25.0%	–	–
Belize	274	–	–	–	–	–
Benin	6,720	37.0%	–	–	–	–
Bhutan	874	–	–	–	–	–
Bolivia	8,814	26.8%	37.6%	19.4%	25+	35.0%
Bosnia and Herzegovina	4,140	37.6%	49.2%	29.7%	18–65	44.9%
Botswana	1,722	21.0%	–	–	–	–
Brazil	176,596	–	21.8%	14.0%	18+	7.7%
Brunei Darussalam	356	20.0%	–	–	–	–
Bulgaria	7,823	32.7%	43.8%	23.0%	16+	52.3%
Burkina Faso	12,109	12.6%	17.7%	0.6%	11–25	–
Burundi	7,206	14.6%	15.6%	11.4%	19+	–
Cambodia	13,404	35.0%	66.7%	10.0%	15+	–
Cameroon	16,087	35.7%	–	–	–	–
Canada	31,630	20.0%	22.0%	17.0%	15+	12.9%
Cape Verde	470	–	–	–	–	–
Central African Rep.	3,881	–	–	–	–	–
Chad	8,582	–	24.1%	–	–	–
Chile	15,774	42.4%	48.3%	36.8%	17+	30.5%
China	1,288,400	–	67.0%	1.9%	18+	26.8%
Colombia	44,584	18.9%	26.8%	11.3%	18–69	25.9%
Comoros	600	–	–	–	–	–
Congo	3,757	7.8%	–	–	–	–
Congo, Dem. Rep.	53,153	–	–	–	–	–
Cook Islands	18	56.8%	34.4%	71.1%	15+	–
Costa Rica	4,005	19.4%	29.0%	9.7%	20–49	19.0%
Côte d'Ivoire	16,835	24.4%	42.3%	1.8%	15+	–
Croatia	4,445	30.3%	34.1%	26.6%	18–65	12.5%
Cuba	11,326	36.8%	48.1%	26.2%	15+	25.0%
Cyprus	770	37.4%	38.5%	7.6%	15+	–
Czech Republic	10,202	25.4%	31.1%	20.1%	15+	22.3%
Denmark	5,387	28.0%	31.0%	25.0%	15+	10.8%
Djibouti	705	42.5%	75.0%	10.0%	13+	–
Dominica	71	–	–	–	–	–

4 Youth smoking prevalence percentages (national data)		5 Passive smoking Youth exposed to passive smoking at home percentages	6 Cigarette consumption annual per person	Countries
male	female			
–	–	–	–	Afghanistan
9.0%	3.2%	85.1%	1,196	Albania
–	–	–	794	Algeria
–	–	–	–	Angola
0.0%	1.1%	18.9%	–	Antigua and Barbuda
16.4%	28.3%	69.9%	1,310	Argentina
–	–	–	1,787	Armenia
24.0%	23.0%	–	1,500	Australia
26.1%	37.1%	–	1,340	Austria
–	–	–	904	Azerbaijan
11.8%	3.0%	39.7%	2,609	Bahrain
–	–	–	243	Bangladesh
3.6%	3.6%	22.0%	513	Barbados
36.2%	27.8%	–	2,160	Belarus
–	–	–	2,566	Belgium
11.4%	5.9%	15.5%	745	Belize
–	–	28.3%	–	Benin
–	–	–	–	Bhutan
–	–	46.6%	250	Bolivia
12.8%	5.4%	96.7%	2,504	Bosnia and Herzegovina
3.2%	2.3%	36.3%	–	Botswana
–	–	39.3%	807	Brazil
–	–	–	–	Brunei Darussalam
31.2%	35.5%	68.5%	3,441	Bulgaria
–	–	38.3%	191	Burkina Faso
–	–	–	95	Burundi
2.4%	0.0%	50.6%	–	Cambodia
–	–	–	471	Cameroon
15.5%	13.5%	–	1,556	Canada
–	–	–	–	Cape Verde
–	–	–	–	Central African Rep.
–	–	–	–	Chad
–	–	57.4%	1,034	Chile
–	–	53.7%	1,771	China
–	–	41.3%	769	Colombia
–	–	–	–	Comoros
–	–	–	–	Congo
–	–	–	113	Congo, Dem. Rep.
24.7%	24.3%	57.2%	–	Cook Islands
–	–	30.0%	–	Costa Rica
–	–	–	192	Côte d'Ivoire
23.2%	24.9%	94.2%	2,015	Croatia
–	–	59.6%	–	Cuba
–	–	–	–	Cyprus
28.7%	30.6%	41.6%	2,445	Czech Republic
16.7%	21.0%	–	1,801	Denmark
8.2%	0.0%	–	–	Djibouti
7.0%	4.3%	28.1%	–	Dominica

Table A **The demographics of tobacco**

Countries	1 Population thousands	2 Adult smoking prevalence				3 Health professionals' smoking prevalence percentages
		percentages			Age span	
		total	male	female	years	
Dominican Republic	8,739	13.4%	15.8%	10.9%	18+	–
Ecuador	13,008	31.1%	45.5%	17.4%	18+	32.4%
Egypt	67,559	28.8%	45.4%	12.1%	20+	–
El Salvador	6,533	25.0%	38.0%	12.0%	18+	7.9%
Equatorial Guinea	494	–	–	–	–	–
Eritrea	4,390	7.2%				–
Estonia	1,353	28.9%	45.0%	17.9%	16–64	13.7%
Ethiopia	68,613	3.1%	5.9%	0.3%	18+	8.8%
Fiji	835	15.0%	26.0%	3.9%	15–85	26.0%
Finland	5,212	22.2%	25.7%	19.3%	15+	6.3%
France	59,762	25.4%	30.0%	21.2%	15+	27.9%
Gabon	1,344	–	–	–	–	–
Gambia	1,421	21.5%	38.5%	4.4%	15+	–
Georgia	5,126	27.8%	53.3%	6.3%	18+	44.2%
Germany	82,541	32.5%	37.3%	28.0%	18+	24.9%
Ghana	20,669	4.1%	7.4%	0.7%	18+	–
Greece	11,033	37.6%	46.8%	29.0%	–	34.3%
Grenada	105	–	–	–	–	–
Guatemala	12,307	11.0%	21.0%	2.0%	13–87	18.0%
Guinea	7,909	57.6%	58.9%	47.3%	11–72	–
Guinea-Bissau	1,489	–	–	–	–	–
Guyana	769	–	–	–	–	–
Haiti	8,440	10.4%	14.6%	6.1%	20+	–
Honduras	6,969	24.0%	36.0%	11.0%	18+	–
Hong Kong SAR	6,816	12.8%	22.0%	3.5%	15+	5.0%
Hungary	10,128	33.8%	40.5%	27.8%	18+	19.3%
Iceland	289	22.4%	25.4%	19.6%	15+	3.6%
India	1,064,399	31.7%	46.6%	16.8%	18+	9.6%
Indonesia	214,674	28.7%	58.3%	2.9%	15+	–
Iran, Isl. Rep.	66,392	10.6%	22.0%	2.1%	15+	34.8%
Iraq	24,700	22.5%	40.0%	5.0%	16+	–
Ireland	3,994	27.0%	28.0%	26.0%	18+	5.0%
Israel	6,688	23.8%	31.9%	17.8%	15+	7.0%
Italy	57,646	24.0%	31.3%	17.2%	15+	28.3%
Jamaica	2,643	22.5%	37.7%	11.6%	25+	–
Japan	127,573	29.6%	46.9%	14.5%	20+	–
Jordan	5,308	29.8%	50.5%	8.3%	18+	27.0%
Kazakhstan	14,878	37.3%	65.3%	9.3%	18+	–
Kenya	31,916	11.2%	21.3%	1.0%	18+	–
Kiribati	96	44.4%	56.5%	32.3%	16+	–
Korea, Dem. People's Rep. of	22,612	42.0%	–	–	–	–
Korea, Republic of	47,912	34.7%	64.9%	4.4%	20+	–
Kuwait	2,396	17.0%	34.4%	1.9%	18–60	18.4%
Kyrgyzstan	5,052	25.4%	51.0%	4.5%	18+	–
Lao People's Dem. Rep.	5,660	–	58.7%	12.5%	18+	17.9%
Latvia	2,321	33.2%	51.1%	19.2%	15–64	–
Lebanon	4,498	35.7%	42.3%	30.6%	25–65	7.0%
Lesotho	1,793	19.8%	38.5%	1.0%	15+	–

4 Youth smoking prevalence percentages (national data)		5 Passive smoking Youth exposed to passive smoking at home percentages	6 Cigarette consumption annual per person	Countries
male	female			
–	–	–	609	Dominican Republic
–	–	35.1%	287	Ecuador
6.3%	2.5%	29.0%	1,414	Egypt
12.7%	3.2%	16.1%	285	El Salvador
–	–	–	–	Equatorial Guinea
–	–	–	–	Eritrea
30.4%	18.2%	81.7%	2,342	Estonia
–	–	16.7%	53	Ethiopia
10.2%	5.3%	51.7%	801	Fiji
28.3%	32.2%	–	1,165	Finland
26.0%	26.7%	–	1,647	France
–	–	–	726	Gabon
–	–	–	–	Gambia
32.7%	8.6%	94.7%	793	Georgia
32.2%	33.7%	–	1,790	Germany
2.6%	1.4%	21.9%	138	Ghana
13.5%	14.1%	–	3,054	Greece
1.8%	1.4%	29.8%	–	Grenada
–	–	30.6%	433	Guatemala
–	–	–	–	Guinea
–	–	–	–	Guinea-Bissau
2.0%	3.5%	34.3%	965	Guyana
–	–	–	–	Haiti
17.1%	13.5%	30.2%	976	Honduras
–	–	–	1,503	Hong Kong SAR
28.2%	25.8%	84.6%	2,296	Hungary
–	–	–	1,769	Iceland
6.6%	1.1%	42.9%	85	India
–	–	67.9%	1,122	Indonesia
2.4%	0.0%	42.9%	807	Iran, Isl. Rep.
–	–	–	–	Iraq
19.5%	20.5%	–	2,159	Ireland
16.9%	11.6%	–	1,905	Israel
21.8%	24.9%	–	2,088	Italy
6.6%	4.2%	30.8%	570	Jamaica
11.0%	5.0%	–	2,920	Japan
16.6%	5.1%	64.8%	1,699	Jordan
14.2%	8.6%	–	1,956	Kazakhstan
7.6%	3.8%	29.5%	235	Kenya
–	–	–	–	Kiribati
–	–	–	–	Korea, Dem. People's Rep. of
–	–	–	2,348	Korea, Republic of
13.1%	3.7%	45.5%	1,362	Kuwait
9.1%	2.7%	–	1,357	Kyrgyzstan
–	–	43.8%	–	Lao People's Dem. Rep.
28.9%	21.1%	60.1%	1,798	Latvia
5.8%	2.2%	79.6%	–	Lebanon
11.4%	5.0%	44.6%	–	Lesotho

101

Table A The demographics of tobacco

Countries	1 Population thousands	2 Adult smoking prevalence percentages			Age span years	3 Health professionals' smoking prevalence percentages
		total	male	female		
Liberia	3,374	–	–	–	–	–
Libyan Arab Jamahiriya	5,559	4.0%	–	–	–	–
Lithuania	3,454	28.3%	43.7%	12.8%	20–64	13.3%
Luxembourg	448	33.0%	39.0%	26.0%	15+	4.5%
Macedonia, Former Yugos. Rep. of	2,049	36.0%	40.0%	32.0%	15+	33.7%
Madagascar	16,894	–	–	–	–	–
Malawi	10,962	–	20.5%	4.8%	18+	–
Malaysia	24,774	–	43.0%	1.6%	18+	10.6%
Maldives	293	–	37.4%	15.6%	–	–
Mali	11,652	–	–	–	–	–
Malta	399	23.4%	29.9%	17.6%	15+	8.7%
Marshall Islands	53	–	–	–	–	–
Mauritania	2,848	–	–	–	–	–
Mauritius	1,222	16.6%	32.1%	1.0%	18+	–
Mexico	102,291	8.8%	12.9%	4.7%	18+	19.0%
Micronesia, Federated States of	125	–	42.0%	–	–	–
Moldova, Republic of	4,238	15.7%	33.6%	1.8%	15+	–
Monaco	33	–	–	–	–	–
Mongolia	2,480	30.0%	52.4%	7.5%	35+	5.0%
Morocco	30,113	14.3%	28.5%	0.1%	18+	16.9%
Mozambique	18,791	–	–	–	–	–
Myanmar	49,363	24.3%	36.4%	12.2%	18+	–
Namibia	2,015	16.2%	22.8%	9.6%	18+	–
Nauru	10	54.4%	49.8%	59.0%	25+	–
Nepal	24,660	36.3%	48.5%	24.0%	18+	–
Netherlands	16,222	32.0%	35.8%	28.4%	15+	–
New Zealand	4,009	–	23.7%	22.2%	15+	–
Nicaragua	5,480	–	–	5.3%	–	–
Niger	11,762	35.1%	40.6%	11.3%	15–35	–
Nigeria	136,461	8.9%	15.4%	0.5%	15+	5.0%
Niue	2	26.1%	37.5%	14.5%	15+	–
Norway	4,562	26.0%	27.2%	24.8%	16–74	7.7%
Oman	2,599	8.6%	15.5%	1.5%	15+	–
Pakistan	148,439	16.0%	28.5%	3.4%	15+	32.0%
Palau	20	–	14.0%	4.0%	20+	–
Palestinian Authority	3,367	22.0%	40.7%	3.2%	adult	26.4%
Panama	2,984	12.9%	19.7%	6.1%	15+	10.4%
Papua New Guinea	5,502	37.0%	46.0%	28.0%	15+	–
Paraguay	5,643	15.1%	23.4%	6.8%	18+	31.7%
Peru	27,148	33.8%	52.5%	17.8%	20–49	25.7%
Philippines	81,503	24.1%	40.5%	7.6%	18+	22.1%
Poland	38,196	32.0%	40.0%	25.0%	15+	14.8%
Portugal	10,444	20.5%	32.8%	9.5%	15+	–
Qatar	624	–	37.0%	0.5%	adults	4.6%
Romania	21,744	20.8%	32.3%	10.1%	15+	43.2%
Russian Federation	143,425	35.1%	60.4%	15.5%	18+	–
Rwanda	8,395	–	7.0%	4.0%	40+	–
Saint Kitts and Nevis	47	–	–	–	–	–

4 Youth smoking prevalence percentages (national data)		5 Passive smoking Youth exposed to passive smoking at home percentages	6 Cigarette consumption annual per person	Countries
male	female			
–	–	–	–	Liberia
2.0%	0.5%	40.3%	–	Libyan Arab Jamahiriya
34.9%	17.9%	48.2%	1,767	Lithuania
–	–	–	–	Luxembourg
14.6%	12.7%	91.6%	2,417	Macedonia, Former Yugos. Rep. of
–	–	–	372	Madagascar
–	–	18.7%	124	Malawi
–	–	–	1,246	Malaysia
–	–	–	–	Maldives
–	–	60.5%	–	Mali
16.9%	17.4%	–	–	Malta
–	–	–	–	Marshall Islands
16.1%	4.7%	47.6%	–	Mauritania
20.8%	6.8%	–	1,319	Mauritius
–	–	38.8%	733	Mexico
–	–	50.5%	–	Micronesia, Federated States of
19.4%	5.2%	–	–	Moldova, Republic of
–	–	–	–	Monaco
14.3%	5.1%	–	–	Mongolia
3.1%	0.4%	27.7%	733	Morocco
–	–	26.7%	–	Mozambique
24.8%	2.8%	53.7%	–	Myanmar
–	–	–	–	Namibia
–	–	–	–	Nauru
4.9%	1.3%	37.8%	488	Nepal
22.5%	24.3%	–	2,392	Netherlands
–	–	–	979	New Zealand
18.6%	5.9%	–	639	Nicaragua
12.6%	6.0%	44.9%	–	Niger
–	–	34.8%	179	Nigeria
–	–	–	–	Niue
20.1%	26.6%	–	698	Norway
3.7%	1.9%	21.8%	–	Oman
0.7%	0.1%	–	618	Pakistan
–	–	46.0%	–	Palau
–	–	60.1%	–	Palestinian Authority
7.6%	10.1%	30.9%	474	Panama
–	–	–	–	Papua New Guinea
–	–	40.4%	–	Paraguay
–	–	29.0%	167	Peru
10.0%	2.9%	60.1%	1,478	Philippines
19.3%	12.6%	68.3%	2,371	Poland
17.6%	26.2%	–	2,125	Portugal
–	–	–	–	Qatar
–	–	89.4%	2,018	Romania
27.4%	18.5%	45.8%	2,792	Russian Federation
–	–	–	–	Rwanda
1.4%	0.7%	17.5%	–	Saint Kitts and Nevis

Table A The demographics of tobacco

Countries	1 Population thousands	2 Adult smoking prevalence				3 Health professionals' smoking prevalence percentages
		percentages			Age span	
		total	male	female	years	
Saint Lucia	161	19.9%	37.3%	5.6%	25+	–
Saint Vincent and Grenadines	109	8.6%	17.4%	1.9%	19+	–
Samoa	178	42.0%	60.0%	24.0%	29+	–
San Marino	28	22.7%	28.0%	17.0%	14+	–
Sao Tome and Principe	157	44.1%	–	–	–	–
Saudi Arabia	22,528	9.3%	14.4%	4.9%	30+	20.0%
Senegal	10,240	32.0%	–	–	–	27.6%
Serbia and Montenegro	8,104	40.4%	48.0%	33.6%	–	18.1%
Seychelles	84	–	37.0%	6.9%	12–64	–
Sierra Leone	5,337	21.5%	40.8%	7.4%	15+	–
Singapore	4,250	13.7%	24.2%	3.5%	18–64	–
Slovakia	5,390	32.0%	41.1%	14.7%	15+	–
Slovenia	1,995	23.7%	28.0%	20.1%	15–64	7.4%
Solomon Islands	457	–	–	23.0%	15+	–
Somalia	9,626	–	–	–	–	–
South Africa	45,829	15.5%	23.2%	7.7%	18+	19.0%
Spain	41,101	31.7%	39.2%	24.6%	16+	34.7%
Sri Lanka	19,232	12.5%	23.2%	1.7%	18+	–
Sudan	33,546	12.5%	23.5%	1.5%	adult	–
Suriname	438	–	–	–	–	–
Swaziland	1,106	6.7%	10.5%	2.9%	18+	–
Sweden	8,956	17.5%	16.7%	18.3%	16–84	6.0%
Switzerland	7,350	24.6%	26.5%	23.1%	15+	8.8%
Syrian Arab Republic	17,384	25.0%	44.3%	5.7%	25–41	–
Tajikistan	6,305	–	–	–	–	–
Tanzania, United Republic of	35,889	25.5%	23.0%	1.3%	25–64	–
Thailand	62,014	25.7%	48.5%	2.9%	15+	2.4%
Timor-Leste	877	–	–	1.1%	20+	–
Togo	4,861	–	–	–	–	–
Tonga	102	31.7%	52.9%	10.5%	15+	–
Trinidad and Tobago	1,313	23.3%	42.4%	4.2%	35–74	–
Tunisia	9,895	26.0%	49.5%	2.4%	18+	–
Turkey	70,712	31.2%	49.4%	17.6%	15+	41.6%
Turkmenistan	4,864	14.0%	27.0%	1.0%	18+	–
Tuvalu	10	41.0%	51.0%	31.0%	20+	–
Uganda	25,280	14.3%	25.2%	3.3%	–	2.8%
Ukraine	48,356	31.8%	52.5%	11.1%	18+	–
United Arab Emirates	4,041	9.3%	17.3%	1.3%	18+	–
United Kingdom	59,329	26.0%	27.0%	25.0%	16+	3.5%
United States of America	290,810	21.6%	24.1%	19.2%	18+	3.3%
Uruguay	3,380	29.2%	34.6%	23.8%	18+	27.0%
Uzbekistan	25,590	12.5%	24.1%	0.9%	–	–
Vanuatu	210	27.1%	49.1%	5.0%	20+	–
Venezuela	25,674	28.7%	35.9%	21.4%	20–89	10.8%
Viet Nam	81,314	18.5%	35.3%	1.7%	18+	–
Yemen	19,173	53.0%	77.0%	29.0%	adult	–
Zambia	10,744	8.5%	16.0%	1.0%	–	–
Zimbabwe	11,635	11.1%	20.0%	2.2%	18+	–

4 Youth smoking prevalence percentages (national data)		5 Passive smoking Youth exposed to passive smoking at home	6 Cigarette consumption annual per person	Countries
male	female	percentages		
4.3%	0.4%	27.4%	–	Saint Lucia
5.1%	2.6%	32.5%	–	Saint Vincent and Grenadines
–	–	–	–	Samoa
–	–	–	–	San Marino
–	–	–	–	Sao Tome and Principe
3.3%	–	30.6%	917	Saudi Arabia
7.9%	1.5%	45.9%	344	Senegal
–	–	–	1,927	Serbia and Montenegro
16.0%	10.8%	43.8%	–	Seychelles
–	–	–	–	Sierra Leone
11.3%	7.7%	36.1%	–	Singapore
31.3%	27.1%	79.0%	1,813	Slovakia
27.9%	30.2%	68.1%	2,631	Slovenia
–	–	–	–	Solomon Islands
–	–	–	–	Somalia
14.8%	8.3%	–	771	South Africa
23.6%	32.3%	–	2,831	Spain
1.7%	0.7%	51.3%	303	Sri Lanka
9.8%	0.3%	30.5%	–	Sudan
11.0%	3.3%	57.2%	–	Suriname
–	–	31.8%	–	Swaziland
11.1%	19.0%	–	1,501	Sweden
25.4%	24.1%	–	2,718	Switzerland
7.3%	2.7%	54.2%	1,161	Syrian Arab Republic
–	–	–	–	Tajikistan
5.9%	2.2%	–	200	Tanzania, United Republic of
–	–	–	813	Thailand
–	–	–	–	Timor-Leste
7.4%	1.4%	28.3%	339	Togo
–	–	–	–	Tonga
9.1%	1.6%	38.0%	–	Trinidad and Tobago
14.5%	1.1%	62.8%	1,865	Tunisia
11.2%	3.1%	–	1,373	Turkey
–	–	–	–	Turkmenistan
–	–	–	–	Tuvalu
–	–	28.7%	154	Uganda
44.6%	22.8%	49.9%	1,389	Ukraine
8.6%	1.0%	31.6%	–	United Arab Emirates
–	–	–	1,380	United Kingdom
17.5%	12.3%	42.1%	1,886	United States of America
–	–	62.6%	1,204	Uruguay
–	–	–	443	Uzbekistan
–	–	–	–	Vanuatu
5.4%	5.8%	42.4%	645	Venezuela
–	–	60.3%	1,230	Viet Nam
4.0%	1.7%	40.2%	577	Yemen
–	–	30.5%	–	Zambia
–	–	35.6%	439	Zimbabwe

Table B The business of tobacco

Countries	1 Growing tobacco			2 Tobacco trade			
	Land devoted to growing tobacco hectares	Agricultural land devoted to tobacco farming percentage of total	Tobacco produced thousands of metric tonnes	Cigarette exports millions	Cigarette imports millions	Tobacco leaf exports metric tonnes	Tobacco leaf imports metric tonnes
Afghanistan	–	–	–	–	–	–	–
Albania	2,500	0.2018%	2.8	31	11,383	1,837	44
Algeria	5,500	0.0135%	5.7	7	0	–	10,476
Angola	3,500	0.0061%	3.3	–	–	–	118
Antigua and Barbuda	–	–	–	–	–	–	6
Argentina	66,000	0.0373%	118.0	131	1	78,437	1,567
Armenia	1,000	0.0638%	3.0	493	2,604	221	1,452
Australia	3,000	0.0007%	9.0	1,220	1,646	2,299	22,100
Austria	100	0.0034%	0.2	40,274	3,599	1,494	25,945
Azerbaijan	2,100	0.0333%	6.5	1,344	1,259	4,991	4,389
Bahrain	–	–	–	52	1,303	–	36
Bangladesh	33,000	0.3362%	40.0	–	935	4,554	6,712
Barbados	–	–	–	35	191	–	5
Belarus	800	0.0090%	1.4	1,207	6,699	16	8,527
Belgium	376	0.0287%	1.2	4616	–	63,012	71,855
Belize	–	–	–	0	29	–	1
Benin	1,300	0.0320%	1.0	422	–	–	14
Bhutan	110	0.0190%	0.2	–	–	–	1
Bolivia	1,060	0.0029%	1.0	143	79	20	137
Bosnia and Herzegovina	3,100	0.1554%	4.0	187	3,345	846	2,576
Botswana	–	–	–	–	1	28	99
Brazil	469,678	0.1305%	928.3	2,871	42	465,981	10,802
Brunei Darussalam	–	–	–	–	89	–	15
Bulgaria	40,000	0.7393%	60.0	3,223	50	25,401	10,576
Burkina Faso	1,000	0.0096%	0.5	33	–	72	93
Burundi	970	0.0445%	0.8	97	–	163	79
Cambodia	9,685	0.1607%	7.4	297	15,246	249	1,999
Cameroon	3,400	0.0371%	4.5	51	383	205	80
Canada	17,000	0.0281%	48.0	3,258	710	21,341	6,447
Cape Verde	–	–	–	1	–	–	–
Central African Rep.	600	0.0117%	0.5	18	–	–	–
Chad	145	0.0003%	0.2	–	–	20	7
Chile	2,970	0.0149%	9.3	2,559	201	1,384	1,858
China	1,352,000	0.2402%	2409.5	19,153	25,706	183,701	64,335
Colombia	13,000	0.0293%	28.0	14,963	4,386	6,585	7,329
Comoros	–	–	–	–	–	–	41
Congo	8,000	0.0027%	0.1	–	–	929	83
Congo, Dem. Rep.	280	0.0353%	3.7	–	2,261	336	954
Cook Islands	–	–	–	–	0	–	–
Costa Rica	117	0.0041%	0.2	3	1,377	93	1,065
Côte d'Ivoire	20,000	0.1005%	10.2	30	870	206	2,290
Croatia	5,394	0.1746%	10.2	7,506	49	5,306	4,219
Cuba	33,942	0.5100%	34.5	335	–	5,995	205
Cyprus	80	0.0658%	0.4	4,544	3,225	300	–
Czech Republic	–	–	–	9,278	7,401	405	16,244
Denmark	–	–	–	5,787	1,030	1,020	15,963
Djibouti	–	–	–	–	–	–	2,969
Dominica	–	–	–	6	3	–	20

Number of cigarette-manufacturing workers per 10,000 workers	Cigarettes manufactured millions	Marlboro or equivalent international brand $US per pack	Local brand	Tax as a proportion of cigarette price	Signed	Ratified	Tobacco industry documents on the Legacy website	Countries
–	–	–	–	–	Jun–04	–	23	Afghanistan
26.4	–	–	–	58.0%	Jun–04	–	39	Albania
64.7	16,826	3.46	–	–	Jun–03	–	98	Algeria
–	–	1.90	0.65	–	Jun–04	–	48	Angola
–	–	–	–	–	Jun–04	–	20	Antigua and Barbuda
38.9	36,500	0.99	1.02	70.0%	Sep–03	–	3,061	Argentina
–	2,815	–	–	–	–	Nov–04	38	Armenia
16.7	22,842	6.68	5.99	67.9%	Dec–03	Oct–04	18,458	Australia
47.5	36,748	5.25	4.80	75.4%	Aug–03	Sep–05	5,078	Austria
34.7	5,550	1.33	0.71	–	–	Nov–05	41	Azerbaijan
0.0	–	1.45	–	40.5%	–	–	371	Bahrain
24.8	20,344	1.18	0.63	65.0%	Jun–03	Jun–04	198	Bangladesh
–	–	–	–	–	Jun–04	Nov–05	82	Barbados
–	10,524	–	–	–	Jun–04	Sep–05	64	Belarus
60.9	13,100	5.13	4.68	75.0%	Jan–04	Nov–05	4,262	Belgium
–	–	–	–	–	Sep–03	–	13	Belize
–	–	–	–	–	Jun–04	Nov–05	19	Benin
–	–	–	–	–	Dec–03	Aug–04	2	Bhutan
6.2	1,436	–	–	39.6%	Feb–04	Sep–05	383	Bolivia
52.1	5,000	–	–	55.0%	–	–	17	Bosnia and Herzegovina
0.0	–	–	–	–	Jun–03	Jan–05	74	Botswana
25.9	96,705	1.04	0.91	65.6%	Jun–03	Nov–05	7,655	Brazil
–	–	1.85	1.23	–	Jun–04	Jun–04	132	Brunei Darussalam
280.4	–	2.57	0.42	64.4%	Dec–03	Nov–05	525	Bulgaria
3.8	–	–	–	45.5%	Dec–03	–	39	Burkina Faso
–	–	–	–	–	Jun–03	–	10	Burundi
23.0	–	1.00	–	–	May–04	–	44	Cambodia
7.4	–	2.44	2.52	19.7%	May–04	–	75	Cameroon
15.2	37,937	7.26	6.11	76.3%	Jul–03	Nov–04	23,357	Canada
32.9	–	–	–	–	Feb–04	Oct–05	3	Cape Verde
–	–	–	–	–	Dec–03	Nov–05	1	Central African Rep.
–	–	–	–	–	Jun–04	–	197	Chad
8.0	13,800	2.23	1.71	76.4%	Sep–03	Jun–05	2,174	Chile
30.2	1,793,423	1.67	1.23	38.0%	Nov–03	Oct–05	7,158	China
5.4	33,010	1.18	0.71	–	–	–	1,130	Colombia
–	–	–	–	–	Feb–04	–	3	Comoros
–	–	–	–	–	Mar–04	–	39	Congo
–	–	–	–	–	Jun–04	Oct–05	–	Congo, Dem. Rep.
–	–	–	–	–	May–04	May–04	7	Cook Islands
14.7	–	1.21	0.91	–	Jul–03	–	950	Costa Rica
9.4	700	2.42	1.21	36.0%	Jul–03	–	107	Côte d'Ivoire
52.2	15,047	3.10	2.23	71.1%	Jun–04	–	114	Croatia
–	–	–	–	–	Jun–04	–	298	Cuba
80.3	–	4.91	–	72.1%	May–04	Oct–05	590	Cyprus
36.1	24,700	2.60	2.10	67.3%	Jun–03	–	2,040	Czech Republic
46.4	12,039	5.60	5.60	76.1%	Jun–03	Dec–04	3,113	Denmark
–	–	–	–	–	May–04	Jul–05	35	Djibouti
–	–	–	–	–	Jun–04	–	42	Dominica

Table B **The business of tobacco**

Countries	1 Growing tobacco			2 Tobacco trade			
	Land devoted to growing tobacco hectares	Agricultural land devoted to tobacco farming percentage of total	Tobacco produced thousands of metric tonnes	Cigarette exports millions	Cigarette imports millions	Tobacco leaf exports metric tonnes	Tobacco leaf imports metric tonnes
Dominican Republic	14,000	0.3788%	18.0	–	26	2,980	6,928
Ecuador	4,300	0.0516%	8.0	13	141	1,077	381
Egypt	–	–	–	65	5	–	64,168
El Salvador	600	0.0352%	1.1	0	1,442	–	409
Equatorial Guinea	–	–	–	–	–	–	–
Eritrea	–	–	–	–	–	–	–
Estonia	–	–	–	81	2,296	–	–
Ethiopia	4,500	0.0147%	3.0	–	–	–	844
Fiji	350	0.0587%	0.4	7	14	–	93
Finland	–	–	–	298	1,965	–	2,372
France	8,451	0.0301%	24.3	17,570	53,520	27,416	75,106
Gabon	–	–	–	9	108	–	670
Gambia	–	–	–	24	334	–	370
Georgia	900	0.0331%	1.5	348	1,717	112	2,139
Germany	5,000	0.0282%	12.0	131,601	32,623	50,585	195,289
Ghana	3,950	0.0269%	1.4	724	–	396	220
Greece	56,006	0.7049%	121.0	19,504	10,977	80,831	22,131
Grenada	–	–	–	2	63	–	22
Guatemala	9,232	0.2048%	20.5	1,959	705	3,283	1,059
Guinea	2,000	0.0163%	1.8	83	–	23	12
Guinea–Bissau	–	–	–	–	–	–	25
Guyana	100	0.0057%	0.1	2	506	–	–
Haiti	450	0.0264%	0.5	–	–	–	641
Honduras	1,170	0.3951%	5.2	4,330	472	1,957	5,512
Hong Kong SAR	–	–	–	6,373	–	760	8,192
Hungary	5,500	0.0934%	9.0	400	473	4,047	8,609
Iceland	–	–	–	–	348	–	10
India	438,000	0.1794%	598.0	1,690	271	120,637	1,029
Indonesia	145,000	0.3725%	141.0	27,784	33	40,639	29,579
Iran, Isl. Rep.	20,000	0.0344%	21.0	0	23,968	7,409	3,500
Iraq	–	–	–	–	–	–	–
Ireland	–	–	–	123	2,168	30	7,343
Israel	0	0	0.0	16	5,292	–	3,183
Italy	36,500	0.2440%	102.8	109	59,367	120,883	52,268
Jamaica	1,175	0.2290%	1.8	18	–	–	9
Japan	21,538	0.4439%	52.7	19,907	83,203	2,714	81,931
Jordan	2,900	0.2595%	2.0	9,514	188	107	3,779
Kazakhstan	7,400	0.0036%	16.0	1,152	767	–	–
Kenya	15,000	0.0567%	20.0	1,490	20	5,028	2,228
Kiribati	–	–	–	–	43	–	–
Korea, Dem. People's Rep. of	45,000	1.6364%	64.0	3	1,101	20	1,203
Korea, Republic of	18,000	1.0864%	35.7	34,652	5,702	1,563	33,687
Kuwait	–	–	–	112	–	–	2
Kyrgyzstan	5,330	0.0240%	13.0	–	2,021	14,312	1,446
Lao People's Dem. Rep.	5,720	0.2914%	33.0	–	97	–	1,313
Latvia	–	–	–	1,403	3,447	737	2,536
Lebanon	9,000	2.6748%	10.0	44	9,574	8,389	1,708
Lesotho	–	–	–	–	–	–	–

3 Manufacturing		4 Price		5 Tax	6 WHO FCTC		7 Tobacco industry documents on the Legacy website	Countries
number of cigarette-manufacturing workers per 100,000 workers	Cigarettes manufactured millions	Marlboro or equivalent international brand $US per pack	Local brand	as a proportion of cigarette price	Signed	Ratified		
71.4	3,437	0.81	0.45	–	–	–	416	Dominican Republic
10.5	–	1.90	1.50	–	Mar–04	–	955	Ecuador
77.4	64,971	1.25	1.25	–	Jun–03	Feb–05	1,143	Egypt
0.0	–	–	–	–	Mar–04	–	557	El Salvador
–	–	–	–	–	–	Sep–05	–	Equatorial Guinea
4.5	–	–	–	–	–	–	3	Eritrea
0.0	–	1.87	1.09	71.8%	Jun–04	Jul–05	158	Estonia
2.7	–	0.92	0.23	–	Feb–04	–	35	Ethiopia
32.0	–	–	–	–	Oct–03	Oct–03	113	Fiji
15.0	3,386	5.26	5.07	75.6%	Jun–03	Jan–05	6,512	Finland
17.2	35,533	6.18	5.92	80.4%	Jun–03	Oct–04	9,220	France
9.6	–	–	–	–	Aug–03	–	21	Gabon
0.0	–	–	–	–	Jun–03	–	59	Gambia
–	1,894	1.50	0.35	–	Feb–04	–	3,875	Georgia
31.5	205,200	5.18	4.64	74.5%	Oct–03	Dec–04	14,552	Germany
13.4	–	1.00	0.33	–	Jun–03	Nov–04	84	Ghana
56.1	–	3.29	2.96	73.5%	Jun–03	–	2,051	Greece
–	–	–	–	–	Jun–04	–	36	Grenada
14.4	3,850	1.76	1.57	–	Sep–03	–	1,254	Guatemala
–	–	–	–	–	Apr–04	–	–	Guinea
–	–	–	–	–	–	–	14	Guinea–Bissau
–	–	–	–	–	–	Sep–05	36	Guyana
–	–	–	–	–	Jul–03	–	131	Haiti
169.5	6,010	–	–	–	Jun–04	Feb–05	298	Honduras
31.9	13,865	4.10	4.36	–	–	–	12,173	Hong Kong SAR
43.3	18,100	3.23	2.30	74.1%	Jun–03	Apr–04	1,160	Hungary
0.0	–	9.03	9.03	–	Jun–03	Jun–04	435	Iceland
128.5	54,991	1.53	1.13	72.7%	Sep–03	Feb–04	2,655	India
253.9	–	0.66	0.91	31.0%	–	–	1,330	Indonesia
42.3	–	1.41	0.45	–	Jun–03	Nov–05	426	Iran, Isl. Rep.
29.6	–	–	–	–	Jun–04	–	179	Iraq
59.8	4,552	8.16	8.16	78.4%	Sep–03	Nov–05	10,327	Ireland
28.2	3,486	4.04	2.77	–	Jun–03	Aug–05	6,898	Israel
33.4	–	4.90	3.34	75.2%	Jun–03	–	3,520	Italy
61.8	960	3.83	3.00	–	Sep–03	Jul–05	429	Jamaica
8.7	249,300	2.87	2.58	61.1%	Mar–04	Jun–04	34,428	Japan
55.6	–	1.76	1.13	–	May–04	Aug–04	17,112	Jordan
28.2	25,400	0.55	–	–	Jun–04	–	212	Kazakhstan
10.3	–	1.59	1.06	–	Jun–04	Jun–04	309	Kenya
–	–	–	–	–	Apr–04	Sep–05	–	Kiribati
–	–	–	–	–	Jun–03	Apr–05	30	Korea, Dem. People's Rep. of
11.2	122,341	2.48	1.59	–	Jul–03	May–05	3,621	Korea, Republic of
0.0	–	1.62	–	29.0%	Jun–03	–	873	Kuwait
102.9	2,927	–	–	–	Feb–04	–	11	Kyrgyzstan
33.2	–	–	–	–	Jun–04	–	93	Lao People's Dem. Rep.
28.8	2,434	–	–	60.3%	May–04	Feb–05	112	Latvia
108.0	–	–	–	–	Mar–04	–	1,113	Lebanon
–	–	–	–	–	Jun–04	Jan–05	23	Lesotho

Table B **The business of tobacco**

Countries	1 Growing tobacco			2 Tobacco trade			
	Land devoted to growing tobacco hectares	Agricultural land devoted to tobacco farming percentage of total	Tobacco produced thousands of metric tonnes	Cigarette exports millions	Cigarette imports millions	Tobacco leaf exports metric tonnes	Tobacco leaf imports metric tonnes
Liberia	–	–	–	–	224	–	315
Libyan Arab Jamahiriya	700	0.0045%	1.6	–	274	–	110
Lithuania	–	–	–	3,626	1,016	79	2,926
Luxembourg	0	0	0.0	7,377	5,836	272	7,864
Macedonia, Former Yugos. Rep. of	17,716	1.6586%	21.1	1,219	232	22,687	3,531
Madagascar	1,900	0.0069%	1.3	7	9	18	235
Malawi	122,000	2.8446%	69.5	2	269	107,031	202
Malaysia	11,000	0.1271%	13.9	12,327	2,079	1,704	17,634
Maldives	–	–	–	–	227	–	31
Mali	824	0.0028%	1.0	1	–	154	4
Malta	–	–	–	908	–	5	5
Marshall Islands	–	–	–	–	–	–	–
Mauritania	–	–	–	–	–	–	565
Mauritius	350	0.3106%	0.5	117	251	–	11
Mexico	11,461	0.0116%	21.9	3,944	2,964	9,032	22,287
Micronesia, Federated States of	–	–	–	–	–	–	–
Moldova, Republic of	10,000	0.3646%	10.2	20	2,083	8,549	2,415
Monaco	–	–	–	–	–	–	–
Mongolia	–	–	–	8	923	–	–
Morocco	2,400	0.0165%	4.0	4	2,818	487	6,687
Mozambique	8,500	0.0145%	12.0	–	–	11,363	27
Myanmar	26,000	0.2348%	49.0	–	–	–	632
Namibia	–	–	–	272	257	–	88
Nauru	–	–	–	–	–	–	–
Nepal	3,398	0.0758%	3.3	–	37	–	3,931
Netherlands	–	–	–	103,277	17,030	18,927	109,700
New Zealand	0	0	0.0	408	215	19	3,832
Nicaragua	1,395	0.0186%	2.2	4	2,070	1,638	243
Niger	1,000	0.0061%	1.0	799	2,427	20	7
Nigeria	22,000	0.0319%	9.2	–	13,396	10	5,789
Niue	–	–	–	–	–	–	–
Norway	–	–	–	22	1,650	163	6,241
Oman	270	0.0247%	1.3	13,789	17,362	114	228
Pakistan	46,800	0.1818%	83.7	163	20	4,111	24
Palau	–	–	–	–	–	–	–
Palestinian Authority	305	0.0709%	0.2	–	–	5	400
Panama	1,250	0.0529%	2.3	2	1,069	5	8
Papua New Guinea	–	–	–	12	2	134	459
Paraguay	8,268	0.0215%	16.5	3,452	–	4,736	19,252
Peru	1,050	0.0023%	12.2	604	565	131	280
Philippines	33,771	0.3355%	47.8	6,691	5,975	10,810	23,509
Poland	10,300	0.0561%	22.0	12,518	5	6,275	19,248
Portugal	2,100	0.0459%	5.5	7,103	2,373	5,240	11,788
Qatar	–	–	–	4	1,298	–	12
Romania	5,830	0.0613%	7.5	1,129	5,623	1,389	20,758
Russian Federation	220	0.0002%	0.1	6,875	4,313	2,743	280,721
Rwanda	2,800	0.1514%	3.8	7	–	–	153
Saint Kitts and Nevis	–	–	–	–	–	–	–

Number of cigarette-manufacturing workers per 10,000 workers	Cigarettes manufactured (millions)	Marlboro or equivalent international brand $US per pack	Local brand	Tax as a proportion of cigarette price	Signed	Ratified	Tobacco industry documents on the Legacy website	Countries
3 Manufacturing		4 Price		5 Tax	6 WHO FCTC		7	
–	–	–	–	–	Jun–04	–	124	Liberia
–	–	–	–	–	Jun–04	Jun–05	46	Libyan Arab Jamahiriya
26.5	7,618	1.39	0.41	60.9%	Sep–03	Dec–04	169	Lithuania
–	–	4.08	3.47	69.0%	Jun–03	Jun–05	767	Luxembourg
625.8	–	–	–	48.3%	–	–	903	Macedonia, Former Yugos. Rep. of
–	–	–	–	–	Sep–03	Sep–04	16	Madagascar
0.0	–	–	–	–	–	–	595	Malawi
91.8	27,163	1.42	1.26	–	Sep–03	Sep–05	2,965	Malaysia
–	–	–	–	75.0%	May–04	May–04	7	Maldives
–	–	–	–	–	Sep–03	Oct–05	42	Mali
107.3	–	3.55	–	76.1%	Jun–03	Sep–03	265	Malta
–	–	–	–	–	Jun–03	Dec–04	603	Marshall Islands
–	–	–	–	–	Jun–04	Oct–05	30	Mauritania
24.2	–	–	–	–	Jun–03	May–04	84	Mauritius
13.0	48,850	1.63	1.45	–	Aug–03	May–04	4,989	Mexico
–	–	–	–	–	Jun–04	Mar–05	82	Micronesia, Federated States of
119.1	6,310	0.80	–	–	Jun–04	–	59	Moldova, Republic of
–	–	–	–	–	–	–	1,525	Monaco
0.0	–	–	–	–	Jun–03	Jan–04	20	Mongolia
19.5	12,216	3.52	0.88	72.8%	Apr–04	–	299	Morocco
2.3	–	–	–	–	Jun–03	–	48	Mozambique
7.6	–	–	–	75.0%	Oct–03	Apr–04	632	Myanmar
0.0	–	–	–	–	Jan–04	Nov–05	21	Namibia
–	–	–	–	–	–	Jun–04	4	Nauru
25.0	–	1.01	0.67	24.7%	Dec–03	–	65	Nepal
72.6	115,561	5.13	4.80	73.1%	Jun–03	Jan–05	2,954	Netherlands
24.1	2,648	7.28	7.04	69.5%	Jun–03	Jan–04	4,969	New Zealand
–	–	–	–	–	Jun–04	–	319	Nicaragua
–	–	–	–	–	Jun–04	Aug–05	171	Niger
–	–	1.50	1.19	–	Jun–04	Oct–05	718	Nigeria
–	–	–	–	–	Jun–04	Jun–05	5	Niue
–	825	10.29	10.29	–	Jun–03	Jun–03	4,000	Norway
0.0	–	–	–	40.5%	–	Mar–05	232	Oman
12.6	55,318	1.10	0.81	–	May–04	Nov–04	953	Pakistan
–	–	–	–	–	Jun–03	Feb–04	20	Palau
–	–	–	–	–	–	–	118	Palestinian Authority
0.0	–	1.20	1.20	–	Sep–03	Aug–04	2,137	Panama
–	–	2.30	2.30	–	Jun–04	–	104	Papua New Guinea
109.4	–	0.71	0.48	–	Jun–03	–	349	Paraguay
–	–	1.69	1.53	–	Apr–04	Nov–04	866	Peru
35.3	75,916	0.69	0.46	–	Sep–03	Jun–05	3,296	Philippines
47.0	81,500	2.26	1.69	72.3%	Jun–04	–	3,308	Poland
23.3	25,261	3.09	2.89	77.6%	Jan–04	Nov–05	978	Portugal
–	–	–	–	40.1%	Jun–03	Jul–04	170	Qatar
40.1	30,000	1.24	0.91	71.7%	Jun–04	–	349	Romania
28.9	–	1.50	0.85	32.9%	–	–	1,556	Russian Federation
–	–	–	–	–	Jun–04	Oct–05	4	Rwanda
–	–	–	–	–	Jun–04	–	20	Saint Kitts and Nevis

Table B **The business of tobacco**

Countries	1 Growing tobacco			2 Tobacco trade			
	Land devoted to growing tobacco hectares	Agricultural land devoted to tobacco farming percentage of total	Tobacco produced thousands of metric tonnes	Cigarette exports millions	Cigarette imports millions	Tobacco leaf exports metric tonnes	Tobacco lea imports metric tonne
Saint Lucia	–	–	–	1	100	–	9
Saint Vincent and Grenadines	70	0.4375%	0.1	0	–	–	18
Samoa	40	0.0305%	0.1	–	–	–	-
San Marino	–	–	–	–	–	–	-
Sao Tome and Principe	–	–	–	–	31	–	-
Saudi Arabia	–	–	–	50	13,340	20	400
Senegal	0	0	0.0	1,125	50	167	3,98:
Serbia and Montenegro	6,800	0.2016%	10.0	222	–	2,535	4,87;
Seychelles	–	–	–	19	37	–	3;
Sierra Leone	40	0.0014%	<0.1	12	–	11	42;
Singapore	0	0	0.0	16,473	13,021	192	13,85(
Slovakia	935	0.0452%	1.3	1,039	4,233	2,266	2,89:
Slovenia	–	–	–	3,162	1,950	531	4,12(
Solomon Islands	100	0.0870%	0.1	–	46	–	15(
Somalia	–	–	–	–	–	–	(
South Africa	12,000	0.0141%	31.9	15,410	307	16,399	30,07
Spain	12,400	0.0385%	33.7	3,915	47,041	30,899	27,24(
Sri Lanka	3,075	0.1337%	3.8	156	115	1,648	3,24:
Sudan	–	–	–	–	–	28	83:
Suriname	–	–	–	6	–	–	3(
Swaziland	200	0.0144%	0.1	50	–	–	42;
Sweden	0	0	0.0	303	11,423	5	3,05;
Switzerland	635	0.0445%	1.2	23,174	295	6,614	30,56:
Syrian Arab Republic	16,000	0.1149%	26.5	79	2,420	2,435	(
Tajikistan	3,200	0.0752%	7.2	–	–	1,922	2(
Tanzania, United Republic of	34,000	0.0848%	24.5	149	18	22,583	86
Thailand	39,500	0.2055%	80.0	419	7,597	33,849	3,66(
Timor–Leste	0	0	0.0	–	–	–	(
Togo	4,000	0.1102%	1.8	78	1,783	114	(
Tonga	–	–	–	–	62	–	(
Trinidad and Tobago	120	0.0752%	0.2	1,694	24	–	2,46(
Tunisia	2,300	0.0298%	2.3	1,782	2,333	398	6,99(
Turkey	183,954	0.4581%	160.0	8,971	1	113,711	48,93(
Turkmenistan	1,600	0.0049%	3.0	–	–	–	2(
Tuvalu	–	–	–	–	–	–	(
Uganda	15,000	0.1218%	33.0	271	137	7,710	53(
Ukraine	3,000	0.0041%	4.0	3,605	–	1,860	66,30(
United Arab Emirates	30	0.0084%	1.3	–	26,872	690	89(
United Kingdom	–	–	–	50,415	8,402	12,285	78,95(
United States of America	165,130	0.0421%	398.8	121,403	23,085	156,894	261,10(
Uruguay	900	0.0057%	3.0	3,605	29	219	2,91(
Uzbekistan	6,700	0.0248%	19.0	150	531	9,698	44(
Vanuatu	–	–	–	–	–	–	(
Venezuela	3,246	0.0149%	6.1	2,717	21	884	6,05(
Viet Nam	18,800	0.2789%	27.4	–	–	5,145	32,33(
Yemen	5,500	0.0306%	11.9	3	96	160	17,49(
Zambia	4,500	0.0128%	4.8	0	–	4,704	44(
Zimbabwe	40,000	0.3918%	80.0	1,395	–	135,405	4,06(

3 Manufacturing		4 Price		5 Tax	6 WHO FCTC		7 Tobacco	Countries
mber of cigarette-manufacturing workers per 00,000 workers	Cigarettes manufactured millions	Marlboro or equivalent international brand $US per pack	Local brand	as a proportion of cigarette price	Signed	Ratified	industry documents on the Legacy website	
–	–	–	–	–	Jun–04	Nov–05	12	Saint Lucia
–	–	–	–	–	Jun–04	–	536	Saint Vincent and Grenadines
–	–	–	–	–	Sep–03	Nov–05	51	Samoa
–	–	–	–	–	Sep–03	Jul–04	7	San Marino
–	–	–	–	–	Jun–04	–	1	Sao Tome and Principe
–	–	1.47	–	50.3%	Jun–04	May–05	2,685	Saudi Arabia
6.1	–	1.15	0.43	–	Jun–03	Jan–05	212	Senegal
83.9	–	1.56	0.49	61.0%	Jun–04	–	71	Serbia and Montenegro
–	–	–	–	–	Sep–03	Nov–03	17	Seychelles
–	–	–	–	–	–	–	51	Sierra Leone
–	–	5.86	5.37	–	Dec–03	May–04	3,227	Singapore
–	–	2.46	2.11	62.0%	Dec–03	May–04	57	Slovakia
–	5,662	2.91	2.35	74.2%	Sep–03	Mar–05	98	Slovenia
–	–	–	–	–	Jun–04	Aug–04	10	Solomon Islands
–	–	–	–	–	–	–	66	Somalia
11.2	35,700	2.65	2.53	46.2%	Jun–03	Apr–05	1,256	South Africa
42.0	60,500	3.42	2.37	71.4%	Jun–03	Jan–05	5,005	Spain
256.1	4,765	2.01	1.80	76.7%	Sep–03	Nov–03	117	Sri Lanka
–	–	1.93	–	–	Jun–04	Oct–05	185	Sudan
–	–	–	–	–	Jun–04	–	22	Suriname
–	–	–	–	–	Jun–04	–	51	Swaziland
23.4	2,310	5.64	5.49	69.6%	Jun–03	Jul–05	4,988	Sweden
–	37,160	4.70	4.70	63.3%	Jun–04	–	6,925	Switzerland
251.8	–	–	–	–	Jul–03	Nov–04	117	Syrian Arab Republic
13.5	585	–	–	–	–	–	10	Tajikistan
33.6	4,850	1.11	0.83	–	Jan–04	–	142	Tanzania, United Republic of
32.9	30,772	1.43	0.99	60.0%	Jun–03	Nov–04	3,413	Thailand
–	–	–	–	–	May–04	Dec–04	3	Timor–Leste
–	–	1.15	0.77	–	May–04	–	33	Togo
0.0	–	–	–	–	Sep–03	Apr–05	10	Tonga
44.5	2,432	–	–	–	Aug–03	Aug–04	315	Trinidad and Tobago
63.6	13,230	2.56	1.30	–	Aug–03	–	119	Tunisia
60.0	–	2.86	2.38	77.0%	Apr–04	Dec–04	2,593	Turkey
–	–	–	–	–	–	–	7	Turkmenistan
–	–	–	–	–	Jun–04	Sep–05	–	Tuvalu
5.7	–	–	–	–	Mar–04	–	63	Uganda
23.8	–	0.76	0.61	–	Jun–04	–	435	Ukraine
–	–	1.63	1.50	31.9%	Jun–04	Nov–05	374	United Arab Emirates
21.7	107,922	9.37	9.02	78.0%	Jun–03	Dec–04	25,398	United Kingdom
18.3	500,000	4.41	4.04	27.0%	May–04	Nov–05	1,252,304	United States of America
26.9	6,296	5.07	1.17	59.0%	Jun–03	Sep–04	669	Uruguay
–	6,519	1.17	–	–	–	–	81	Uzbekistan
–	–	–	–	–	Apr–04	Sep–05	3	Vanuatu
18.5	13,500	0.90	0.86	–	Sep–03	–	2,108	Venezuela
31.6	74,580	1.27	0.57	37.3%	Sep–03	Dec–04	977	Viet Nam
21.3	5,780	–	–	–	Jun–03	–	77	Yemen
13.5	–	2.00	0.78	–	–	–	136	Zambia
58.1	–	1.16	1.16	–	–	–	1,425	Zimbabwe

113

SOURCES

Please note that some figures in tables and graphs throughout the atlas may not appear to sum due to rounding.

In the sources below op. cit. is used to refer to identical citations in the same numbered section.

PART ONE PREVALENCE AND HEALTH

Part-title quote
Chapman Simon. Blaming tobacco's victims. *Tobacco Control* 2002;11(3):167-168.

1 Types of tobacco use

Map
Gupta PC. Survey of socio-demographic characteristics of tobacco use among 99,598 individuals in Bombay, India using hand-held computers. *Tobacco Control* 1996;5(2):114–20.
WHO. *Tobacco or Health: A Global Status Report*. Geneva: WHO. 1997.
WHO. *Guidelines for controlling and monitoring the tobacco epidemic*. Geneva: WHO. 1998.

Roll-your-own cigarettes
Darrall KG & Figgins JA. Roll-your-own smoke yields: theoretical and practical aspects. *Tobacco Control* 1998;7(2):168–75.
De Stefani E, Barrios E, Fierro L. Black (air-cured) and blond (flue-cured) tobacco and cancer risk III: oesophageal cancer. *European Journal of Cancer* 1993;29A:763–6. 4.
De Stefani E, Oreggia F, et al. Hand-rolled cigarette smoking and risk of cancer of the mouth, pharynx and larynx. *Cancer* 1992;70:679–82.
Tuyns AJ, Esteve J. Pipe, commercial and hand-rolled cigarette smoking in oesophageal cancer. *International Journal of Epidemiology* 1983;12:110–3.

2 Male smoking

Text
Ezzati M, Lopez AD. Estimates of global mortality attributable to smoking in 2000. *Lancet* 2003 Sep 13;362(9387):847–52.
Scull R. Bright Future Predicted for Asia Pacific. *World Tobacco*. Sept 1986:35.

Smoking prevalence for men
The specific age ranges vary for different countries, and are given in the tables.
WHO Global InfoBase team. *The SuRF Report 2. Surveillance of chronic disease risk factors: Country-level data and comparable estimates*. Geneva: WHO. 2005.
WHO WPRO.
http://www.wpro.who.int/information_sources/databases/regional_statistics/rstat_tobacco_use.htm
http://www.wpro.who.int/health_topics/tobacco
http://www.wpro.who.int/media_centre/fact_sheets/fs_20020528.htm Accessed 04 August 2005.
WHO EURO. Tobacco Free Initiative. Tobacco Control Database.
http://data.euro.who.int/tobacco Accessed July 2005.
Afghanistan – Wielgosz AT. WHO assignment Afghanistan noncommunicable diseases CVD 1991.
Albania – *Evaluation of smoking prevalence among adult population*. November 2001. Institute of Public Health. Downloaded from WHO EURO Tobacco Control Database .
Algeria – République Algérienne Démocratique et Populaire Ministère de la Santé et al. Mesure des facteurs de risque des maladies non transmissibles dans deux zones pilotes (approche STEPWISE) *Algérie 2003-Rapport*. 2004.
American Samoa – Mishra SI, Osann K, Luce PH. Prevalence and predictors of smoking behavior among Samoans in three geographical regions. *Ethnicity & Disease* 2005 Spring; 15(2):305–15.
Andorra –Health for All database. WHO EURO Tobacco Control Database .

Argentina – Virolini M (Ministerio de Salud). *Encuesta Nacional de Tabaco 2004*. Ministerio de Salud y Ambiente de la Nacion.
Armenia – Gilmore A et al. Prevalence of Smoking in 8 countries of the Former Soviet Union: Results from the Living Conditions, Lifestyles and Health Study. *American Journal of Public Health* 2004. 94:2177–87.
Australia – Australian Institute of Health and Welfare 2005. *2004 National Drug Strategy Household Survey: First Results*. AIHW cat. no. PHE 57. Canberra: AIHW (Drug Statistics Series No. 13). Accessed 27 Sept 2005.
http://www.aihw.gov.au/publications/phe/ndshs04/ndshs04.pdf
Austria – Ulmer H et al. Recent trends and sociodemographic distribution of cardiovascular risk factors: results from two population surveys in the Austrian WHO CINDI demonstration area. *Wiener klinische Wochenschrift.*. 2001. 113:573–9. Additional data from personal communication: Hanno Ulmer, Institute of Biostatistics, University of Innsbruck.
Azerbaijan – Adventist Development and Relief Agency et al. *Reproductive Health Survey*. Azerbaijan. 2001. Atlanta, U. S. Department of Health and Human Services, 2003.
Bahamas – PAHO. *Tobacco or Health: Status in the Americas Pan American Health Organization*. 1992.
Bahrain – State of Bahrain. *The 2001 census of population, housing, buildings and establishments*. 2002.
Bangladesh – WHO World Health Survey.
Barbados – Cooper R et al. The prevalence of hypertension in seven populations of West African origin. *American Journal of Public Health*. 1997. 87:160–8. Additional data from personal communication: Richard Cooper.
Belarus – Health for All database. WHO EURO Tobacco Control Database .
Belgium – Health for All database WHO EURO Tobacco Control Database .
Benin – Fourn L and Monteiro B. Smoking and health in Benin. *World Health Forum* 1988;9:589–90.
Bolivia – Barceló A et al. Diabetes in Bolivia. *Pan American Journal of Public Health* 2001;10:318–23. Additional data from personal communication: Alberto Barceló.
Bosnia and Herzegovina – Noncommunicable disease risk factor survey: Federation of Bosnia and Herzegovina 2002; Ministry of Health of Bosnia and Herzegovina, Public Health Institute of Bosnia and Herzegovina. Downloaded from WHO EURO Tobacco Control Database .
Botswana – WHO. *Tobacco or health: a global status report*. Geneva. 1997.
Brazil – WHO. World Health Survey.
Brunei Darussalam – Tobacco-Free Initiative Western Pacific Region. *Country Profiles on Tobacco or Health 2000*. WHO. WPR 2000. http://www.wpro.who.int
Bulgaria – *Health Interview Survey*. National Statistical Institute. WHO EURO Tobacco Control Database .
Burkina Faso – Sondo B et al. Tabagisme des élèves dans établissements secondaires du Burkina Faso. *Revue des Maladies Resporatoires* 1996;13:493-497.
Burundi – Mahwenya P. Analyse de la situation actuelle du tabagisme au Burundi. 1998.
Cambodia – National Institute of Statistics. *Cambodian Socioeconomic Survey 1999*. Phnom Penh: Author.
Cameroon – Cameroon smoking population. (2000). TMA – International Tobacco Guide (ITG). [CD-ROM]. Princeton, NJ: Author. http://www.tma.org/tma/products/Compendiums/itg.htm
Canada – *Canadian Tobacco Use Monitoring Survey Annual 2004*. http://www.hc-sc.gc.ca/hl-vs/pubs/tobac-tabac/ctums-esutc-

2004/tabl01_e.html Accessed 23 Sept 2005.
Chad – Leonard L. Cigarette smoking and perceptions about smoking and health in Chad. *East African Medical Journal* 1996;73:509–12.
Chile – Ministerio de Salud de Chile. *Encuesta Nacional de Salud, Chile 2003*. Chile 2004.
China – China WHO WPRO database. Smoking Statistics. http://www.wpro.who.int/media_centre/fact_sheets/fs_20020528.htm Accessed 28 August 2005.
Colombia –Ministerio de Salud. *II Estudio Nacional de Factores de Riesgo de Enfermedades Cronicas*. Information provided by WHO PAHO Regional Office: 29 April 2003.
Congo – Kimbally-Kaky G et al. *Hypertension arterielle et les autres facteurs de risque cardiovasculaires à Brazzaville*. Brazzaville, Congo; 2004.
Cook Islands – Tobacco-Free Initiative Western Pacific Region. *Country Profiles on Tobacco or Health 2000*. WHO, WPRO, 2000. www.who.int
Costa Rica –Bejarano, J and Ugalde, F (2003). *Estudio Nacional sobre consumo de drogas 2000-2001*. San José: I. A. F. A. Information provided by WHO PAHO Regional Office; 29 April 2003.
Cote D'ivoire –Schmidt, D, et al. En quete sur la consommation tabagique en milieu africain a Abidjan. *Poumon-Coeur* 1981;37: 87-94.
Croatia – *First Croatian Health Project, Sub-project on health promotion, the magnitude and context of problems – Baseline parameters*. Report, Zagreb. WHO EURO Tobacco Control Database .
Cuba – Perez V et al. *National Survey of Risk Factors – 1995*. National Institute of Hygiene, Epidemiology and Microbiology, Ministry of Health and National Statistic Office; 1995.
Cyprus – *A household survey on smoking prevalence and behaviour in Cyprus*. Ministry of Health, Cyprus, 1997. WHO EURO Tobacco Control Database .
Czech Republic – National Institute of Public Health. WHO EURO Tobacco Control Database .
Denmark –WHO Health for All. WHO EURO Tobacco Control Database .
Djibouti –Estimates made by Dr. Abdillahi Hassan Hersi of the Ministry of Health in the unpublished report *Tobacco Related Problems in Djibouti*, submitted 4 July 1999.
Dominican Republic – WHO. World Health Survey.
Ecuador –Ockene, JK, Chiriboga, DE and Zevallos, JC. Smoking in Ecuador: prevalence, knowledge, and attitudes. *Tobacco Control* 1996;5:121–6.
Egypt – Herman WH et al. Diabetes mellitus in Egypt: risk factors and prevalence. *Diabetic Medicine*, 1995;12:1126–31. Additional data from personal communication: William Herman, MD, MPH.
El Salvador – PAHO. *Tobacco or Health: Status in the Americas* 1992.
Eritrea – Ministry of Health, Eritrea. National noncommunicable disease (NCD) risk factor baseline survey (using WHO STEPSwise approach).
Estonia – Health behaviour among the Estonian adult population (part of the international FinBalt Health Monitor survey – Finland, Estonia, Latvia, Lithuania). WHO EURO Tobacco Control Database .
Ethiopia – WHO. World Health Survey.
Fiji – Pryor J (FSM) et al. *Fiji NCD STEPS Report* (Draft) V4. 9.
Finland –Health for All database. WHO EURO Tobacco Control Database .
France – Health for All database. WHO EURO Tobacco Control Database .
Gambia – van der Sande MAB et al. Blood pressure patterns and cardiovascular risk factors in rural and urban Gambian communities. *Journal of Human Hypertension*, 2000;14:489–96. Additional data from personal communication: Marianne AB van der Sande.
Georgia – Prevalence of Smoking in 8 Countries of

the Former Soviet Union: Results from the Living Conditions, Lifestyles and Health Study. *American Journal of Public Health* 2004;94(12):2177–87. WHO EURO Tobacco Control Database .

Germany – Lampert, T and Burger, M. Rauchgewohnheiten in Deutschland – Ergebnisse des telefonischen Bundes-Gesundheitssurveys 2003. *Gesundheitswesen*. 2004;66:511–17. WHO EURO Tobacco Control Database .

Ghana – WHO. World Health Survey.

Greece – Kokkevi, A et al. , *Eur. Addict. Res.* 2000;6(1):42–49. Kokkevi, A et al. *Drug Alcohol Depend.* 2000;58(1–2): 181–188. WHO EURO Tobacco Control Database .

Guam – Centers for Disease Control and Prevention, Prevalence of Current Cigarette Smoking Among Adults and Changes in Prevalence of Current and Some Day Smoking – United States, 1996–2000, *Morbidity and Mortality Weekly Report*. 2003;52;303–7.

Guatemala – Sakhuja R et al. Perceptions and prevalence of smoking among people in the highlands of Guatemala. *Cancer Causes and Control*, 2001;12:479–84.

Guinea –Ngom, A, Dieng, B and Bangoura, M. *Investigation of nicotine addiction in Guinea*. Conakry: Department of Health and Office of WHO in Guinea. 1998.

Haiti – Foundation Haïtienne de Diabète et de Maladies Cardio-Vasculaires. *Prévalence du diabète det de l'hypertension artérielle dans l'aire métropolitaine de Port au Prince, Haïti* (PREDIAH 2003). Haiti, FHADIMAC; 2003.

Honduras – PAHO. *Tobacco or Health: Status in the Americas*, 1992.

Hong Kong – *General Household Survey, 2003*. Hong Kong Department of Health, Available online.

Hungary – WHO Health for All. WHO EURO Tobacco Control Database .

Iceland – WHO Health for All. WHO EURO Tobacco Control Database .

India – WHO World Health Survey.

Indonesia – Soemantri S et al. *National Household Health Survey Morbidity Study: NCD risk factors in Indonesia*. SURKESNAS 2001.

Iran, Islamic Republic of – Azizi F. *Tehran Lipid and Glucose Study*, Endocrine Research Center, Shaheed Beheshti University of Medical Sciences, 2001.

Iraq – WHO. *Tobacco or health: a global status report*. Geneva: WHO; 1997.

Ireland – *The national health & lifestyle surveys 2002*. Health Promotion Unit, Department of Health and Children, 2003. WHO EURO Tobacco Control Database .

Israel – WHO Health for All. WHO EURO Tobacco Control Database .

Italy – WHO Health for All. WHO EURO Tobacco Control Database .

Jamaica – Cooper R et al. The prevalence of hypertension in seven populations of West African origin. *American Journal of Public Health* 1997;87:160–8. Additional data from personal communication: Richard Cooper.

Japan – Higuchi S. *Survey on adult drinking patterns and prevention for related problems*. Ministry of Health, Labour and Welfare, 2004.

Jordan – Shehab F et al. Prevalence of selected risk factors for chronic disease – Jordan, 2002. *Morbidity and Mortality Weekly Report* 2003;52:1042–4.

Kazakhstan – Gilmore A et al. Prevalence of Smoking in 8 countries of the Former Soviet Union: Results from the Living Conditions, Lifestyles and Health Study. *American Journal of Public Health* 2004;94:2177–87.

Kenya – WHO World Health Survey.

Kiribati – Tobacco-Free Initiative Western Pacific Region. *Country Profiles on Tobacco or Health 2000*. WHO, WPRO, 2000. http://www.wpro.who.int

Korea, Democratic People's Republic of – WHO. *Tobacco or health: a global status report*.

Geneva: WHO; 1997. Estimation of smoking in 2000; ERC Statistics International. *The World Cigarette Market*. Suffolk, UK, 2001.

Korea, Republic of – Suh IL. Cardiovascular mortality in Korea: a country experiencing epidemiologic transition. *Acta Cardiologica* 2001;56:75–81.

Kuwait – Memon A et al. Epidemiology of smoking among Kuwaiti adults: prevalence, characteristics, and attitudes. *Bulletin of the WHO*, 2000;78:1306–15.

Kyrgyzstan – Prevalence of Smoking in 8 Countries of the Former Soviet Union: Results from the Living Conditions, Lifestyles and Health Study. *American Journal of Public Health* 2004;94(12): 2177–87. WHO EURO Tobacco Control Database .

Lao People's Democratic Republic – WHO World Health Survey.

Latvia – Health Behaviour among Latvian adult population, 2002. WHO EURO Tobacco Control Database .

Lebanon – Soweid RA et al. *Together for heart health. An initiative for community-based cardiovascular disease risk factor prevention and control*. Nahhal Est 2002. Additional data from personal communication: Prof. Mustafa Khogali.

Lesotho – WHO *Tobacco or health: a global status report*. Geneva: WHO; 1997.

Libyan Arab Jamahiriya – General Secretary of Health and Social Welfare. *Tobacco Control in Libya*. 1997. Annual Report of the Center for Information and Documentation. Libyan Arab Jamahiriya.

Lithuania – Health behaviour among the Lithuanian adult population (part of the international FinBalt Health Monitor survey) WHO EURO Tobacco Control Database .

Luxembourg –WHO Health for All. WHO EURO Tobacco Control Database .

Macedonia, Former Yugoslav Republic of – WHO EURO Tobacco Control Database .

Malawi – WHO World Health Survey.

Malaysia – WHO World Health Survey.

Maldives –*Smoking Survey 2001*. Department of Public Health Malé; 2001.

Malta –Health for All database, WHO EURO Tobacco Control Database .

Mauritius – WHO World Health Survey.

Mexico – WHO World Health Survey.

Micronesia, Federated States of – Shmulewitz D. Epidemiology and factor analysis of obesity, type II diabetes, hypertension, and dyslipidemia (Syndrome X) on the Island of Kosrae, Federated States of Micronesia. *Human Heredity* 2001;51:8–19.

Moldova, Republic of – WHO EURO Tobacco Control Database .

Mongolia – Suvd J et al. Glucose intolerance and associated factors in Mongolia: results of a national survey. *Diabetic Medicine* 2002;19:502–8.

Morocco – WHO World Health Survey.

Myanmar – WHO World Health Survey.

Namibia – WHO World Health Survey.

Nauru – Shaw J. Unpublished data for Nauru. 2003.

Nepal – WHO World Health Survey.

Netherlands –Health for All Database. WHO EURO Tobacco Control Database .

Netherlands Antilles – *Curaçao Health Survey, 1993–94*, http://www.paho.org/english/sha/prflner.htm Accessed 24 July 2005.

New Zealand – *A portrait of health – key results of the 2002/03 New Zealand Health Survey*. Wellington, Ministry of Health; 2004. Additional data from personal communication: Ministry of Health, New Zealand.

Nicaragua – Instituto Nacional de Estadísticas y Censos (INEC) et al. Encuesta Nicaragüense de demografía y salud 2001. Programa DHS+ and ORC Macro; 2002. Additional data from personal

communication: Noureddine Abderrahim of ORC Macro.

Niger – Ministère Jeunesse Sports et Culture et al. Le tabagisme chez les jeunes au Niger. 1990.

Nigeria – **Males:** The National Expert Committee on NCD. Non-communicable diseases in Nigeria. Final report of a national survey. Federal Ministry of Health and Social Services; 1997. **Females:** National Population Commission (NPC) [Nigeria] and ORC Marco. *Nigeria: Demographic and Health Survey 2003*. Calverton, Maryland, National Population Commission and ORC Macro; 2004.

Niue – Laugesen M. *Mission report on tobacco from Niue* 2003. Personal communication: Harley Stanton.

Norway – Interview survey, Statistics Norway; 2004. WHO EURO Tobacco Control Database .

Oman – Sulaiman AJM et al. Oman family health survey 1995. *Journal of Tropical Pediatrics* 2001;47:1–33.

Pakistan – Pakistan Medical Research Council. *National Health Survey of Pakistan 1990–94* Network for the Rational use of Medication in Pakistan; 1998. Additional data from personal communication: A. Q. Khan of Pakistan Medical Research Council.

Palau –Palau Substance Abuse Needs Assessment (SANA) 1998.

Palestinian Authority – Smoking data from the Palestine Central Bureau of Statistics; Reported in *Country Profiles on Tobacco Control in the Eastern Mediterranean Region*. http://www.emro.who.int/TFI/CountryProfile.htm

Panama – Acción Latinoamericana Contra el Cáncer. 1998. Information provided by WHO PAHO Regional Office; 29 April 2003.

Papua New Guinea – Tobacco-Free Initiative Western Pacific Region. Country Profiles on Tobacco or Health 2000. WHO, Western Pacific Regional Office; 2000. http://www.wpro.who.int

Paraguay – WHO. World Health Survey.

Peru – *Encuesta Nacional Sobre Prevención y Uso de Drogas – Informe General, Perú 1999* – Instituto Nacional de Estadística e Informática – Contradrogas (Comisión de Lucha Contra el consumo de Drogas). Information provided by PAHO Regional Office 20 April 2003.

Philippines – WHO World Health Survey.

Poland – Nationwide survey on smoking behaviours and attitudes in Poland; 2000–2002. WHO EURO Tobacco Control Database .

Portugal –WHO Health for All, WHO EURO Tobacco Control Database .

Puerto Rico – "Do you smoke cigarettes now?"; Centers for Disease Control and Prevention. Behavioral Risk Factor Surveillance System. http://apps. nccd. cdc. gov/brfss.

Qatar – Smoking data from the Hamad Medical Center Survey; Reported in *Country Profiles on Tobacco Control in the Eastern Mediterranean Region*. http://www.emro.who.int/TFI/CountryProfile.htm

Romania – *Health Status of population in Romania*, Bucharest 2001, National Institute of Statistics. WHO EURO Tobacco Control Database .

Russian Federation – Anna Gilmore et al. Prevalence of Smoking in 8 Countries of the Former Soviet Union: Results from the Living Conditions, Lifestyles and Health Study. *American Journal of Public Health* 2004;94(12): 2177–87. WHO EURO Tobacco Control Database .

Rwanda – Currently smoking 5 or more cigarettes per day, two main hospitals of Butare; Newton R et al. Cancer in Rwanda. *International Journal of Cancer* 1996;66(1):75–81.

Saint Lucia – Cooper R et al. The prevalence of hypertension in seven populations of West African origin. *American Journal of Public Health* 1997;87:160–8. Additional data from personal communication: Richard Cooper.

Saint Vincent And Grenadines – Ministry of

Health. Risk factor survey in St. Vincent. In: Pan American Health Organization/WHO; 1997.

Samoa – McGarvey ST. Cardiovascular disease (CVD) risk factors in Samoa and American Samoa; 1990-95. *Pacific Health Dialog* 2001;8:157–62. Additional data from personal communication: Stephen McGarvey.

San Marino – Current smoking in the early 1990s: *Tobacco or health: a global status report*. Geneva: WHO; 1997.

Sao Tome And Principe – Smoking at least one cigarette per day (survey year unknown); *Analise da Situacao do Tabagismo em S. Tome E Principe*. Organizacao Mundial da Saude, S. Tome; 1998.

Saudi Arabia – Saudi Heart Association. National cross-sectional study on coronary artery disease risk factors in Saudi Arabia (the CADIS study). 2001. Personal communication: Mansour Al-Nozha, Professor of Medicine and Consultant Cardiologist, Director, King Fahd Cardiac Centre.

Senegal – Kane A et al. Etude épidémiologique des maladies cardiovasculaires et des facteurs de risque en milieu rural au Sénégal. *Cardiologie Tropicale* 1998;25:103–7.

Serbia & Montenegro – Institute of Public Health of Serbia "Dr Milan Jovanovic-Batut". *Health status, health needs and health care in Serbia*, Belgrade 2001 (WHO Survey). WHO EURO Tobacco Control Database .

Seychelles – Bovet P et al. The Seychelles Heart Study II: methods and basic findings. *Seychelles Medical and Dental Journal* 1997;5(1):8–24.

Sierra Leone – Lisk DR et al. Blood Pressure and hypertension in rural and urban Sierra Leoneans. *Ethnicity & Disease* 1999;9:254–63.

Singapore – *National Health Surveillance Survey 2001*. Ministry of Health; 2002.

Slovakia – WHO Health for All, WHO EURO Tobacco Control Database .

Slovenia – Zakotnik-Mavcec J et al. WHO EURO Tobacco Control Database .

Solomon Islands – Tobacco-Free Initiative Western Pacific Region. Country Profiles on Tobacco or Health 2000. WHO. WPRO; 2000. http://www.wpro.who.int

South Africa – WHO. World Health Survey.

Spain – National health survey 2001 (unpublished), Ministry of Health and Consumer Affairs. WHO EURO Tobacco Control Database .

Sri Lanka – WHO World Health Survey.

Sudan – Smoking; Reported in *Country Profiles on Tobacco Control in the Eastern Mediterranean Region*. http://www.emro.who.int/TFI/CountryProfile.htm

Swaziland – WHO World Health Survey.

Sweden – WHO Health for All. WHO EURO Tobacco Control Database .

Switzerland – Office fédéral de la statistique. Enquête suisse sur la santé. 2003. Additional data from personal communication: Marilina Galati-Petrecca, Division santè droit, èducation et science, Section de la santé.

Syrian Arab Republic – Maziak W et al. Smoking behaviour among schoolteachers in the north of the Syrian Arab Republic. *Eastern Mediterranean Health Journal* 2000;6:352–8.

Tanzania, United Republic of – Bovet P et al. Distribution of blood pressure, body mass index and smoking habits in the urban population of Dar es Salaam, Tanzania, and associations with socioeconomic status. *International Journal of Epidemiology* 2002;31:240–7.

Thailand – National Statistical Office et al. *The cigarette smoking and alcoholic drinking behavior survey 2001*. Bangkok, Thailand, National Statistical Office; 2002.

Timor-Leste – Estimated daily smoking; Barraclough S. Women and tobacco in Indonesia. *Tobacco Control* 1999;8: 327-332.

Tokelau – Reported in WHO WPRO Country Profiles, Tobacco or Health 2000. http://www.wpro.who.int

Tonga – Colagiuri S et al. The prevalence of diabetes in the Kingdom of Tonga. *Diabetes Care* 2002;25:1378–83.

Trinidad And Tobago – Miller GJ et al. Adult male all-cause, cardiovascular and cerebrovascular mortality in relation to ethnic group, systolic blood pressure and blood glucose concentration in Trinidad, West Indies. *International Journal of Epidemiology* 1988;17:62–9. Additional data from personal communication: George J Miller.

Tunisia – WHO World Health Survey.

Turkey – WHO Health for All, WHO EURO Tobacco Control Database .

Turkmenistan – Piha T et al. Tobacco or health. *World Health Statistics Quarterly* 1993;46:188–94.

Tuvalu – Current smoking; Tuomilehto J. et al. Smoking rates in the Pacific Islands. *Bulletin of the WHO* 1986;64(3): 447–56.

Uganda – Uganda Bureau of Statistics (UBOS) et al. Uganda Demographic and Health Survey 2000–2001. Calverton, Maryland, UBOS and ORC Macro; 2001.

Ukraine – Gilmore A et al. Prevalence of Smoking in 8 countries of the Former Soviet Union: Results from the Living Conditions, Lifestyles and Health Study. *American Journal of Public Health*; 2004;94:2177–87.

United Arab Emirates – WHO World Health Survey.

United Kingdom – *Living in Britain: Results from the 2002 General Household Survey.* (Covering Great Britain only.) Office for National Statistics http://www.statistics.gov.uk/pdfdir/lib0304.pdf

United States Of America – Centers for Disease Control and Prevention. Cigarette smoking among adults – United States, 2003. *Morbidity and Mortality Weekly Reports* 2005;54(20):509-13

Uruguay – WHO World Health Survey.

Uzbekistan – Ministry of Health et al. *Uzbekistan Health Examination Survey 2002* – preliminary report. Calverton, Maryland, ORC Macro; 2003.

Vanuatu – Carlot-Tary M et al. *Vanuatu non-comunicable disease survey report*. Noumea, New Caledonia, Multipress; 1998.

Venezuela – Garcia-Araujo M et al. Factores nutricionales y metabólicos como riesgo de enfermedades cardiovasculares en una población adulta de la ciudad de Maracaibo Estado Zulia, Venezuela. *Investigacion Clinica* 2001;42:23–42.

Viet Nam – WHO. World Health Survey.

Virgin Islands (USA) – Centers for Disease Control and Prevention, State-Specific Prevalence of Current Cigarette Smoking Among Adults – United States; 2003. *Morbidity and Mortality Weekly Report* 2004;5;1.

Yemen – Sanaa University Survey by A. Hadarani. Reported in *Country Profiles on Tobacco Control in the Eastern Mediterranean Region*. http://www.emro.who.int/TFI/CountryProfile.htm

Zambia – Pampel FC. Patterns of tobacco use in the early epidemic stages: Malawi and Zambia; 2000–02. *Am J Public Health* 2005;95(6):1009–15.

Zimbabwe – WHO World Health Survey.

Smoking trends

Japan 1960–2000: Japan Tobacco Annual Reports. 2001–04 from Yumiko Mochizuki-Kobayashi. (The late) Hirayama T, personal communication; 1995.

UK: Tobacco Advisory Council. In Wald N, Nicolaides-Bouman A. *UK Smoking Statistics*. Second edition; 1991.

Basic Facts: One. Smoking statistics. Action on Smoking and Health. Jan 2005. http://www.ash.org.uk/html/factsheets/html/basic01.html. Accessed 30 June 2005.

General Household Survey 2003, London, Office for National Statistics; 2004. http://www.statistics.gov.uk/ghs Table 8.1 http://www.statistics.gov.uk/statbase/ssdataset.asp?vlnk=8821&More=Y. Accessed 05 July 2005.

USA 1965–99: US Department of Health and Human Services, National Health Interview Survey. In *Women and Smoking: A Report of the Surgeon General*, US Department of Health and Human Services, Centers for Disease Control and Prevention, National Center for Chronic Disease Prevention and Health Promotion, Office on Smoking and Health; 2001.

USA: *Morbidity and Mortality Weekly Report, Cigarette smoking among adults – United States* 1999;50 (40): 869–73, 12 Oct 2001;29:642–5, 26 July 2002.

Early Release of Selected Estimates Based on Data From the January-March 2005 National Health Interview Survey. *Prevalence of current smoking among adults aged 18 years and over, by age group and sex. United States, 2004.* http://www.cdc.gov/nchs/data/nhis/early release/200506_08.pdf Accessed 30 June 2005.

Clipboard

Ibison D. Rothmans' joint deal opens heavenly gates. *Window, Hong Kong*; 16 Oct 1992:4.

Wow: China

China 350m: Marlboro makers jump state go-ahead. *South China Morning Post.* Hong Kong. 25 April 2005. Business p1.

3 Female smoking

Quote

Hypotheses Explaining the Sex Mortality Differential. http://66.102.9.104/search?q=cache:xmQZMS-1DyIJ:www.soa.org/library/monographs/Life/M-LI01-1/M-LI01-1_VII.pdf+%22women+who+smoke+like+men+die+like+men%22&hl=en%20target=nw. Accessed 31 July 2005.

Text

Ezzati M, Lopez AD, Rodgers A, Murray CJL (eds), *Smoking and Oral tobacco use, Comparative Quantification of Health Risks, Global and Regional Burden of Disease Attributable to Selected Major Risk Factors*. WHO: Geneva; 2004. http://www.who.int/publications/cra/chapters/volume1/part4/en/index.html

Smoking prevalence for women

Sources as for 2 Smoking prevalence for men – Male smoking.
The specific age ranges vary for different countries, and are given in the tables.

Smoking trends

Sources as for 2 Smoking prevalence for men – Male smoking.

USA: Centers for Disease Control and Prevention. Cigarette smoking among adults – United States; 2003. MMWR *Morb Mortal Wkly Rep.* 2005;53(20):427–31.

Clipboard

The Female Smoker Market, http://tobaccodocuments.org/landman/0337550 3-5510.html, accessed 12 July 2005.

Wow: Women worldwide

Gajalakshmi CK, Jha P, Ransom K, Ngyyen S. Global patterns of smoking and smoking-attributable mortality. In Chaloupka F. (Ed.). *Tobacco control in developing countries.* Oxford: Oxford University Press; 2002. Tables 2.1 and 2.2, p16.

Haglund M, President, International Network of Woman Against Tobacco. INWAT celebrates its 15th Anniversary. 5 April 2005. http://www.inwat.org/pdf/15th_Anniversary.pdf Accessed 1 July 2005.

4 Health professionals

Quote

WHO. *The Role of Health Professionals in Tobacco Control.* http://www.who.int/tobacco/resources/publications/wntd/2005/bookletfinal_20april.pdf Accessed Aug 2005.

Text

Fiore MC, et al. *Treating Tobacco Use and Dependence. Clinical Practice Guideline.* US Department of Health and Human Services, Public Health Service; 2000.

Gorin SS. Predictors of tobacco control among nursing students, *Patient Education & Counseling* 2001;44(3):251–62.

Terasalmi E et al, *Smoking habits of community pharmacists in 12 European countries and their attitudes towards non-smoking work,* WHO; 2001, EUR/01/5025372.

WHO. Code of practice on tobacco control for health professional organizations. Accessed Aug 2005.
http://www.who.int/tobacco/communications/events/codeofpractice/en/

Smoking prevalence among health professionals

Health Professionals are doctors, dentists, nurses, pharmacists, medical, dental, and pharmacy students, health professionals, health science students, anaesthetists.

ASH Scotland. *ASH Scotland Briefing, Smoke-free Legislation around the World.*
http://www.ashscotland.org.uk/ Accessed June 2005.

WHO EMRO. Tobacco Free Initiative, *Country Profiles on Tobacco Control in the Eastern Mediterranean Region.*
http://www.emro.who.int/tfi/countryprofile.htm Accessed June 2005.

ERC Group plc. *World Cigarettes 2, The 2004 Survey.*

WHO EURO. Tobacco Free Initiative, Tobacco Control Database
http://data.euro.who.int/tobacco Accessed June 2005.

National Tobacco Information Online System (NATIONS). http://apps.nccd.cdc.gov/nations Accessed June 2005.

ERC Statistics International. *The World Cigarette Market.* Suffolk, UK; 2001.

PAHO. *Tobacco or Health: Status of the Americas, a report of the Pan American Health Organization.* Washington DC; 1992 (Scientific Publication No. 536).

Albania – Centers for Disease Control and Prevention. Tobacco Use and Cessation Counseling – Global Health Professionals Survey Pilot Study, 10 Countries, 2005. *Morbidity and Mortality Weekly Report* 2005;54(20):505–9.

Algeria – Tessier JF, Nejjari C and Bennani-Othmani M. Smoking in Mediterranean countries: Europe, North Africa and the Middle-East. Results from a co-operative study. *International Journal of Tuberculosis and Lung Disease* 1999;3(10):927–37.

Argentina – Current smoking in 15 hospitals throughout Buenos Aires measured by the Tobacco or Health Commission, Secretariat of Health; Information provided by Diego Leon Perazzo of the Argentine Antitobacco Union.

Armenia – WHO *Health Professionals and Tobacco Control. A Briefing File for the WHO European Region.* http://www.euro.who.int/document/Tob/TOB_Factsheet.pdf Accessed August 2005.

Australia – Current smoking among practitioners both affiliated and unaffiliated with the Royal Australian College of General Practitioners; Young JM and Ward JE. Declining rates of smoking among medical practitioners [letter]. *Medical Journal of Australia* 1997;167(4):232.

Austria – Kössler W, Lanzenberger M and Zwick H. Smoking habits of office-based general practitioners and internists in Austria and their smoking cessation efforts. *Wiener Klinische Wochenschrift* 2002;114(17–18):762–5.

Bahrain – Behbehani NN, Hamadeh RR, Macklai NS. Knowledge of and attitudes towards tobacco control among smoking and non-smoking physicians in 2 Gulf Arab states. *Saudi Medical Journal* 2004;25(5):585–91.

Bangladesh – *see* Albania.

Bolivia – WHO *Tobacco or Health: A Global Status Report.* Geneva: WHO; 1997.

Bosnia and Herzegovina – Hodgetts G, Broers T, Godwin M. Smoking behaviour, knowledge and attitudes among Family Medicine physicians and nurses in Bosnia and Herzegovina. *BMC Family Practice* 2004;5(1):12.

Brazil – Current smokers among medical students from the Federal University of Rio Grande do Sul; Knorst M. et al. *Smoking prevalence among medical students.* (Presented at the American College of Chest Physicians Conference, 2001).

Bulgaria – Regular daily smoking among general practitioners and specialists in primary health care measured by the National Center of Public Health; Information provided by George Kotarov in the WHO European Region's Tobacco Questionnaire 1996/1997.

Canada – Chalmers K, Seguire M, Brown J. Tobacco use and baccalaureate nursing students: a study of their attitudes, beliefs and personal behaviours. *Journal of Advanced Nursing* 2002;40(1):17–24.

Chile – Bello S et al. A national survey on smoking habit among health care workers in Chile. *Revista Medica de Chile* 2004;132(2):223–32.

China – Zhu T et al. A comparison of smoking behaviors among medical and other college students in China. *Health Promotion International* 2004;19(2):189–96.

Colombia – Rosselli D et al. Smoking in Colombian medical schools: the hidden curriculum. *Preventive Medicine* 2001;33(3):170–4.

Costa Rica – Smoking among all active physicians registered with the College of Physicians and Surgeons of Costa Rica, average age 41 years; Grossman DW et al. Smoking: attitudes of Costa Rican physicians and opportunities for intervention. *Bulletin of the WHO* 1999;77(4):315–22.

Croatia – *see* Armenia.

Cuba – Smoking on a daily basis at the time of the survey measured by the National School of Public Health and the Ministry of Public Health; Information provided by Nery Suarez Lugo of the National School of Public Health.

Czech Republic – *see* Armenia.

Denmark – *see* Armenia.

Ecuador – Sanchez P. Lisanti N. (2003 July). [The prevalence of and attitudes toward smoking among physicians in Azuay, Ecuador]. *Pan American Journal of Public Health* 14(1):25-30.

El Salvador – *see* Albania.

Estonia – *see* Armenia.

Ethiopia –Zein ZA. Cigarette smoking among Ethiopian health professionals and students. *New York State Journal of Medicine* 1987;87(8):433–5.

Fiji –WHO *Tobacco or Health: A Global Status Report.* Geneva: WHO; 1997.

Finland – *see* Armenia.

France – *see* Armenia.

Georgia – *see* Armenia.

Germany – Hoch E. Muehlig S. Hofler M. Lieb R. Wittchen HU. How prevalent is smoking and nicotine dependence in primary care in Germany? *Addiction* 2004;99(12):1586–98.

Greece – Livaditis M et al. Sociodemographic and psychological characteristics associated with smoking among Greek medical students. *European Addiction Research* 2001;7(1):24–31.

Guatemala – Current smokers among medical residents of Roosevelt Hospital and San Juan de Dios Hospital; Barnoya J and Glantz S. Knowledge and use of tobacco among Guatemalan physicians. *Cancer Causes and Control* 2002;13(9): 879–81.

Hong Kong – Daily smoking among doctors newly graduated from the University of Hong Kong; Cheng KK and Lam TH. Smoking among doctors in Hong Kong: a message to medical educators. *Medical Education* 1990;24(2):158–63.

Hungary – Sima A, Piko B, Simon T.

Epidemiologic study of the psychological health and risk behaviors of medical students. *Orvosi Hetilap* 2004;145(3):123–9.

Iceland – *see* Armenia.

India – *see* Albania.

Iran, Islamic Republic of – Cigarette smoking among senior medical students at Shiraz University of Medical Sciences; Ahmadi J, Benrazavi L and Ghanizadeh A. Substance abuse among contemporary Iranian medical students and medical patients. *Journal of Nervous and Mental Disease* 2001;189(12):860–1.

Ireland – *see* Armenia.

Israel – *see* Armenia.

Italy – Pizzo AM et al. Italian general practitioners and smoking cessation strategies. *Tumori* 2003;89(3):250–4.

Jordan – Information provided by Dr. Nisreen Abdul-Latif, WHO, EMRO, Tobacco Free Initiative (15 June 2005).

Kuwait – Behbehani NN, Hamadeh RR, Macklai NS. Knowledge of and attitudes towards tobacco control among smoking and non-smoking physicians in 2 Gulf Arab states. *Saudi Medical Journal* 2004;25(5):585–91.

Lao People's Democratic Republic – Survey of current smoking in four hospitals in the Vientiane municipality conducted by Somsamouth K et al; Ministry of Health, Centre of Information & Education for Health. *Tobacco control programs in Lao PDR.* Vientiane; 2000: Author. Reported by Southeast Asia Tobacco Control Alliance and ASH Thailand. Tobacco Country Profile: Laos. http://tobaccofreeasia.net/Menu1/laos/prevalence.htm

Lebanon – (survey year unknown); Tessier JF, Nejjari C and Bennani-Othmani M. Smoking in Mediterranean countries: Europe, North Africa and the Middle-East. Results from a co-operative study. *International Journal of Tuberculosis and Lung Disease* 1999.3(10):927–37.

Lithuania – Malakauskas K, Veryga A, Sakalauskas R. Smoking prevalence among university hospital staff. *Medicina (Kaunas)* 2003;39(3):301–6.

Luxembourg – *see* Armenia.

Macedonia, The former Yugoslav Republic of – *see* Armenia.

Malaysia – Current smoking among clinical-year medical students at Universiti Kebangsaan in Kuala Lumpur; Frisch AS, Kurtz M and Shamsuddin K Knowledge, attitudes and preventive efforts of Malaysian medical students regarding exposure to environmental tobacco and cigarette smoking. *Journal of Adolescence* 1999;22(5):627–34.

Malta – *see* Armenia.

Mexico – Salmeron-Castro J et al. Smoking among health professionals of the Mexican Social Security Institute, Morelos. *Salud Publica de Mexico* 2002;44 (Suppl 1):S67–75.

Mongolia – WHO *Tobacco or Health: A Global Status Report.* Geneva: WHO; 1997.

Morocco – Alaoui Yazidi A et al. Smoking in Casablanca hospitals: knowledge, attitudes and practices. *Revue des Maladies Respiratoires* 2002;19(4):435–42.

Nigeria – Omokhodion FO. Psychosocial problems of pre-clinical students in the University of Ibadan Medical School. *African Journal of Medicine & Medical Sciences* 2003;32(2):135–8.

Norway – *see* Armenia.

Pakistan – Piryani RM, Rizvi N. Smoking habits amongst house physicians working at Jinnah Postgraduate Medical Center, Karachi, Pakistan. *Tropical Doctor* 2004;34(1):44–5.

Palestinian Authority – Daily smoking among doctors, nurses, lab technicians and administrators (average age 30-49 years) in all of the West Bank's nine health districts, average age 30–49 years; Preventive Medicine Department, Palestinian National Authority Ministry of Health. (1999). *Survey of smoking habits at the workplace among employees of the Primary Health Care Directorate.*

Ramallah: Author. Information provided by Dr. Nadim Toubassi, Director of Primary Health Care and Public Health Directorate, 26 Jan 2000.

Panama – Survey of Ministry of Public Health employees in Colon Province; Information provided by PAHO Regional Office, 29 April 2003.

Paraguay –WHO PAHO *Tobacco or Health: Status in the Americas*. Washington, DC: WHO; 1992.

Peru –Asthon LP et al. El médico y el tabaquismo en el Peru. Acta Cancerológica. 1993. Information provided by PAHO Regional Office 29 April 2003.

Philippines – *see* Albania.

Poland – *see* Armenia.

Qatar – Information provided by Dr. Nisreen Abdul-Latif, WHO, EMRO, Tobacco Free Initiative, 15 June 2005.

Romania – *see* Armenia.

Saudi Arabia – Current smokers among staff at Al-Kharj Military Hospital; Siddiqui S and Ogbeide DO. Profile of smoking amongst health staff in a primary care unit at a general hospital in Riyadh, Saudi Arabia. *Saudi Medical Journal* 2001;*22*(12):1101–4.

Senegal – Ndiaye M et al. Smoking habits among physicians in Dakar. *Revue de Pneumologie Clinique* 2001;57(1 Pt 1):7–11.

Serbia and Montenegro – *see* Albania.

Slovenia – *see* Armenia.

South Africa – Current daily smoking and former smoking among 78% of anesthetists practicing in the Durban area (survey year unknown); Callander C. and Rocke DA. Smoking habits and attitudes of Durban metropolitan anesthetists. *South African Medical Journal* 1986;70: 589–91.

Spain – Regular daily smoking among public sector doctors in Madrid; Regional Office of Oncological Coordination. Regional Ministry of Health and Social Services. *Knowledge and attitudes regarding tobacco of public sector doctors in the community of Madrid, Appendix XIV.* Madrid; 1995.

Sweden – *see* Armenia.

Switzerland – *see* Armenia.

Taiwan – Yang MS, Yang MJ, Pan SM. Prevalence and correlates of substance use among clinical nurses in Kaohsiung city. *Kaohsiung Journal of Medical Sciences* 2001;17(5):261–9.

Thailand – Leggat PA et al. Health of dentists in southern Thailand. *International Dental Journal* 2001;51(5):348-52.

Turkey – *see* Armenia.

Uganda – *see* Albania.

United Kingdom (Great Britain and Northern Ireland) – *see* Albania.

United States of America –Nelson DE et al. Trends in cigarette smoking among US physicians and nurses. *JAMA* 1994.271(16): 1273–5.

Uruguay – Current smoking; (Medical doctors) National survey conducted by Dr. Eduardo Bianco. El tabaquismo y el habito de fumar en los medicos. 2001.

Venezuela – Smoking among medical and nursing students in Lara State; Flores-Finizola A et al. Gender influence and major determinants of tobacco addiction among health science students in Lara State, Venezuela. *CVD Prevention: Journal of the World Heart Federation* 2000.3(1): 59–63.

Counselling students
Smoking students
Centers for Disease Control and Prevention, Tobacco Use and Cessation Counseling – Global Health Professionals Survey Pilot Study, 10 Countries, 2005, *Morbidity and Mortality Weekly Report* 2005;54(20).

R J Reynolds
http://www.tobacco.org/ads, select 'Camel'. Accessed 17 Aug 2005.

Clipboard
Tobacco Institute, *Oregon Preemptive Strategy*, April 30 1996; Bates No. TI30639073/9074.

Wow: Chinese physicians
Findings of the 2002 National Prevalence Survey, Dr Yanwei Wu, WHO, WPRO, Personal Communication, Aug 2005.

5 Boys' tobacco use

Quote
http://www.motivatingquotes.com/healthq.htm Accessed 29 April 2005.

Text
http://www.cdc.gov/tobacco/global/GYTS/pdf/globaluse.pdf

Early starters
The GYTS is a collaborative project of WHO/CDC/participating countries (also include Associate Partners when data are used from countries in which they were involved). Analyses of GYTS data are not necessarily endorsed by WHO/CDC/participating countries.
Global Youth Tobacco Survey Collaborating Group. Differences in worldwide tobacco use by gender: findings from the Global Youth Tobacco Survey. *J Sch Health* 2003;73:207–15.
Current GYTS data downloaded from http://www.cdc.gov/tobacco/global/GYTS.htm
Currie C, Roberts C, Morgan A, et al (Eds). *Young people's health in context. Health Behaviour in School-aged Children (HBSC) study: international report from the 2001/2002 survey*. WHO: Geneva 2004. p67.
White V, Hayman J. *Smoking behaviours of Australian secondary students in 2002*. National Drug Strategy Monograph Series 54. Australian Government Department of Health and Ageing; 2004.

Other tobacco products in India
Global Youth Tobacco Survey Collaborating Group. Tobacco use among youth: a cross country comparison. *Tobacco Control* 2002 Sep;11(3):252–70.
http://www.cdc.gov/tobacco/global/gyts/GYTS_factsheets.htm Accessed 25 July 2005.

Clipboard
Reynolds RJ, 1982. Burrows D, NBER Models of Price Sensitivity by Age/Sex, Reynolds RJ Marketing Development Department letter, 6 Oct 1982, Bates Number 513318391.

Wows: India/youth worldwide
GYTS Collaborating Group. op. cit.

6 Girls' tobacco use

Text
GYTS Collaborating Group. Differences in worldwide tobacco use by gender: findings from the Global Youth Tobacco Survey. *J Sch Health* 2003;73:207–15.
Akbartabartoori M, Lean ME, Hankey CR. Relationships between cigarette smoking, body size and body shape. *Int J Obes* 2005 29(2):236-43.
Honjo K, Siegel M. Perceived importance of being thin and smoking initiation among young girls. *Tobacco Control* 2003;12:289–95.

Early starters
Wow: India/youth worldwide
As for 5 Boys' tobacco use.

Reasons why more young women smoke
INWAT Fact Sheets. http://www.inwat.org Accessed 1 July 2005.

Clipboard
http://tobaccodocuments.org/landman/505938010-8013.html .

7 Cigarette consumption

Quote
Wilde, Oscar. *The Picture of Dorian Gray*. Ed: Norman Page. Broadview Press: Orchard Park, NY; 1998.

Text
Economic Research Service, Cigarette consumption continues to slip, *Agricultural Outlook* Jan–Feb 2001.

ERC. *The World Cigarette Market: The 1999 Survey*, ERC Group Plc; 2000.
McGinn AP. The Nicotine Cartel. *World Watch* 1997;10(4):18–27.
Guindon GE & Boisclair D. 2005. Cigarette consumption dataset 1970–2004. Prepared for the American Cancer Society, Aug 2005.

Annual cigarette consumption
Wow: five countries
Guindon GE & Boisclair D. 2005. Cigarette consumption dataset 1970–2004. Prepared for the American Cancer Society, Aug 2005. Sources include:
Shafey O, Dolwick S, Guidon GE, (eds) Tobacco Control Country Profiles 2003. American Cancer Society, Atlanta, GA, USA; 2003. Per capita cigarette consumption figures constructed from production, trade (import and export) and population data.
ERC Statistics International Plc. *The World Cigarette Market: The 2004 survey*. Suffolk, UK; 2004.
ECOWAS *Social and Economic Indicators 1998*, Economic Community of West African States.
Food and Agriculture Organization of the United Nations (FAO). FaoStat Statistical databases. http://apps.fao.org/
Interstate Statistical Committee of the Commonwealth of Independent States. Official Statistics of the countries of the Commonwealth of Independent States, CD-ROM, 2000–5. http://www.unece.org/stats/cisstat/cd-offst.htm
United Nations dataset *World population prospects 1950–2050* (2004 revision), New York, United Nations Population Division; 2005.
United Nations Industrial Commodity Production Statistics Database, 1950–98, CD-ROM. Prepared by the Industrial Statistics Section, Statistics Division, New York, USA; 2005.
United Nations Statistics Division. Commodity Trade Statistics Database (COMTRADE) http://esa.un.org/unsd/pubs
United States Department of Agriculture, Economic Research Service, Tobacco Statistics.2005. http://usda.mannlib.cornell.edu/data-sets/specialty/94012
United States Department of Agriculture, Foreign Agricultural Service. Tobacco: World Markets and Trade. (Various issues) http://www.fas.usda.gov/currwmt.html
United States Department of Agriculture, Foreign Agricultural Service. Attache Reports.(Various issues) http://www.fas.usda.gov/scriptsw/attacherep/default.asp
United States Department of Agriculture, World Cigarette Consumption, selected countries, 1960–95, Tobacco Statistics Stock #94012 Economic Research Service, Table 170; 1996.

Global cigarette consumption
2002 Proctor RN, personal communication, 2001.
Anne Platt McGinn op. cit.
Guindon GE & Boisclair D; 2005 op.cit.

Regions' share of world cigarette sales
ERC. *The World Cigarette Market: The 2004 Survey*. London: ERC Group Plc; 2004.

8 Health risks

Quote
The Health Consequences of Smoking: A Report of the Surgeon General, 2004. http://www.cdc.gov/tobacco/sgr/sgr_2004/pressrelease.htm Accessed 17 Aug 2005.

Text
American Cancer Society. *Child and teen tobacco use*. http://www.cancer.org/docroot/PED/content/PED_10_2X_Child_and_Teen_Tobacco_Use.asp?sitearea=PED. Accessed Aug 2005.
National Geographic News, *Modified tobacco plant removes TNT from soil*, 7 Dec 2001. http://news.nationalgeographic.com/news/2001/

12/1207_TVplantTNT.html. Accessed Aug 2005.

How tobacco use harms you

American Cancer Society (CPSII) in Surgeon General's Report. *Reducing the Health Consequences of Smoking: 25 Years of Progress.* US Dept of Health and Human Services; 1989. Publication No CDC 89-8411.

British Medical Bulletin 1996;52.(1). Published for the British Council by the Royal Society of Medicine Press Limited. Scientific Editors: Sir Richard Doll and Sir John Crofton.

Doll R, Peto R, Wheatley K, Gray R, Sutherland I. Mortality in relation to smoking: 40 years' observation on male British doctors. *British Medical Journal* 1994;309:901–11.

GASP! Inside Story, Comic Company, 1997.

International Agency for Research on Cancer, Tobacco Smoking and Tobacco Smoke (Group 1), Summary of data reported and evaluation. http://www-cie.iarc.fr/htdocs/monographs/vol83/01-smoking.html. Accessed June 2005.

US Department of Health and Human Services. *The Health Consequences of Smoking: A Report of the Surgeon General.* Atlanta, GA: U.S. Department of Health and Human Services, Centers for Disease Control and Prevention, National Center for Chronic Disease Prevention and Health Promotion, Office on Smoking and Health; 2004.

WHO. *The Smoker's Body.* Accessed July 2005 http://www.who.int/tobacco/resources/publications/smokersbody_en_fr.pdf

Health risks due to smoking in pregnancy

British Medical Association, Board of Science and Education, Tobacco Control Resource Centre. *Smoking and Reproductive Life: The impact of smoking on sexual, reproductive, and child health.*

Ernster V, Kaufman K, Nichter M, Samet J, Yoon SY. Women and Tobacco: Moving from policy to action, *Bulletin of the WHO* 2000;78(7):891–901.

Gajalakshmi V, Peto R, Kanaka TS, Jha P, Smoking and mortality from tuberculosis and other diseases in India: retrospective study of 43000 adult male deaths and 35000 controls. *Lancet* 2003;362(9383):507–15.

Deadly chemicals

Tobacco Ingredients in All Brands, Philip Morris. 11 Jan 2001.

American Lung Association of New Hampshire, *Tobacco Facts.* http://www.nhlung.org/tobacco_facts.cfm. Accessed July 2005.

Crawford MA, Balch GI, Mermelstein R and The Tobacco Control Network Writing Group. Responses to tobacco control policies among youth. *Tobacco Control* 2002;11:14–19.

Clipboards

Mellman AJ. 1983. In: *Tobacco Industry Quotes On Nicotine And Addiction From Recently Released Documents,* Campaign for Tobacco-Free Kids, 26 Oct 1999.

7 CEOs of American Tobacco, Brown & Williamson Tobacco Company, Liggett Group, Lorillard Tobacco Company, Philip Morris, RJR Tobacco Company, US Tobacco Company, to House Commerce Committee, USA; 14 April 1994.

Lee PN, 1979. *Tobacco Explained: The truth about the tobacco industry...in its own words,* Action on Smoking and Health. http://www.ash.org.uk/html/conduct/pdfs/tobexp.pdf Accessed July 2005.

Wow: smoking is responsible for ...

WHO Programme on Tobacco or Health. WHO EB77/22.Add1. 15 Nov 1985.

Wow: time ticks away

Zacharias E. 7 simple tips for a healthy, quality, and long life. 31 May 2001. http://www.bouldermedicalcenter.com/Articles/7_simple_tips.htm Accessed Jan 2002.

9 Passive smoking

Quote

Doll R, Peto J. *Asbestos — effects on health exposure to asbestos,* Her Majesty's Stationery Office; 1985.

Text

Action on Smoking and Health Scotland, *Secondhand Smoke Briefing,* Accessed June 2005 and http://www.ashscotland.org.uk/ash/files/ASH%20Scotland%20SHS%20briefing.doc

Allwright S. *Why Ireland needed to act: the impact of environmental tobacco smoke on worker's health.* Luxembourg: *Smokefree Europe*; 2 June 2005.

California Environmental Protection Agency. *Proposed Identification of Environmental Tobacco Smoke as a Toxic Air Contaminant, SRP Version.* http://www.arb.ca.gov/toxics/ets/dreport/june05/bcovertoc1.pdf Accessed July, 2005.

IARC Working Group on the Evaluation of Carcinogenic Risks to Humans. *Tobacco smoke and involuntary smoking.* IARC Monographs on the Evaluation of Carcinogenic Risks to Humans 2004;83:1–1438.

Scientific Committee on Tobacco and Health (SCOTH). *Secondhand smoke: Review of evidence since 1998.* http://www.ash.org.uk/index.php?navState=&getPage=http://www.ash.org.uk/html/passive.php. Accessed July, 2005.

WHO. *International Consultation on Environmental Tobacco Smoke (ETS) and Child Health.* Geneva: WHO/TFI 11–14 Jan 1999; Report No. WHO/NCD/TFI/99.10:6–11.

Domestic danger

Global Youth Tobacco Survey Collaborating Group. *Global Youth Tobacco Survey Country Fact Sheets.* Centers for Disease Control and Prevention. Accessed June, 2005. http://www.cdc.gov/tobacco/Global/gyts/GYTS_factsheets.htm

Deaths caused by passive smoking

Jamrozik K, Estimate of deaths attributable to passive smoking among UK adults: database analysis, *British Medical Journal* 2005;330(7495):812.

Harm caused by passive smoking

Bonita R., Duncan J, Truelsen T, Jackson RT, & Beaglehole R, Passive smoking as well as active smoking increases the risk of acute stroke, *Tobacco Control,* 1999;8:156–60.

California Environmental Protection Agency, op. cit.

IARC Working Group on the Evaluation of Carcinogenic Risks to Humans, op. cit.

WHO. 1999 op. cit.

Clipboard

Tobacco Institute. *Report on Public Smoking Issue Executive Committee,* 10 April 1985. Report No: Bates No. T104820990/1004.

Wow: USA

Centers for Disease Control and Prevention, Annual Smoking-Attributable Mortality, Years of Potential Life Lost, and Productivity Losses – United States, 1997–2001, *Morbidity and Mortality Weekly Report* 2005;54:625–28.

10 Deaths

Text

Action on Smoking and Health, *Tobacco in the developing world, factsheet no: 21,* Aug 2004. http://www.ash.org.uk/html/factsheets/html/fact21.html#_edn5. Accessed July 2005.

California Environmental Protection Agency, *Proposed Identification of Environmental Tobacco Smoke as a Toxic Air Contaminant, SRP Version.* http://www.arb.ca.gov/toxics/ets/dreport/june05/bcovertoc1.pdf Accessed July, 2005.

Centers for Disease Control and Prevention, Annual Smoking-Attributable Mortality, Years of Potential Life Lost, and Productivity Losses – United States, 1997–2001, *Morbidity and Mortality Weekly Report* 2005;54:625–28.

Ezzati M, Lopez AD, Regional, disease specific patterns of smoking-attributable mortality in 2000, *Tobacco Control,* 2004;13:388–95.

Ezzati M, Lopez AD. Estimates of global mortality attributable to smoking in 2000. *Lancet* 2003;362(9387):847–52.

Jamrozik K, Estimate of deaths attributable to passive smoking among UK adults: database analysis, *British Medical Journal* 2005;330(7495):812.

Peto R, Lopez AD. *The future worldwide health effects of current smoking patterns.* In: Koop CE, Pearson CE, Schwarz MR (eds). *Global Health in the 21st Century,* Jossey-Bass, New York; 2000.

Samet JM, Yoon SY (eds), *Women and the Tobacco Epidemic: Challenges for the 21st Century,* WHO, and the Institute for Global Tobacco Control, Johns Hopkins School of Public Health, Geneva; 2001.

WHO, *International Consultation on Environmental Tobacco Smoke (ETS) and Child Health,* Geneva: WHO/TFI;11–14 Jan 1999;Report No. WHO/NCD/TFI/99.10:6–11.

WHO, *Why is tobacco a public health priority?* Accessed July 2005 and http://www.who.int/tobacco/health_priority/en/index.html

WHO, *Women and Tobacco,* Geneva: WHO, 1992:63–66.

Deaths due to smoking

Distribution by disease

Ezzati M, Lopez AD(eds) 2000 op. cit.

Ezzati M, Lopez AD, Rodgers A, Murray CJL (eds), *Smoking and Oral tobacco use, Comparative Quantification of Health Risks, Global and Regional Burden of Disease Attributable to Selected Major Risk Factors,* WHO: Geneva, 2004.

Wow: smokers killed

Peto R, Lopez AD. 2000 op. cit.

Wow: China (men)

Liu BQ et al. Emerging tobacco hazards in China: 1. Retrospective proportional mortality study of one million deaths. *British Medical Journal* 1998;317:1411–22.

Wow: China (women)

Quan Gan et al. Estimating the Burden of Disease from Passive Smoking in China in 2002. 10th International Conference on Indoor Air Quality and Climate in Beijing, China, 5 Sept 2005.

Wow: India (men)

Gajalakshmi V, Peto R, Kanaka TS & Jha P, Smoking and mortality from tuberculosis and other diseases in India: retrospective study of 43,000 adult male deaths and 35,000 controls. *Lancet,* 2003;362:507–15.

WHO, *Why is tobacco a public health priority?* Accessed July 2005 http://www.who.int/tobacco/health_priority/en/index.html

PART TWO THE COSTS OF TOBACCO

Part-title quote

WHO: *Tobacco and Poverty: A Vicious Cycle,* Geneva: WHO 2004

11 Costs to the ecomomy

Quote

Donald Behan, Fellow of the Society of Actuaries (SOA). Secondhand Smoke Costs U.S. Economy $10 Billion Annually, According to New Study by Society of Actuaries, PR Newswire, 17 Aug 2005. Accessed 12 Sept 2005 http://www.mindfully.org/Health/2005/Secondhand-Smoke-Cost17aug05.htm

Text

WHO, Tobacco Free Initiative. Framework Convention on Tobacco Control. http://www.who.int/tobacco/framework/fctc_booklet_english.pdf Accessed June 2005.

Economic costs

Alcohol Advisory Council of New Zealand. The Social costs of Tobacco Use and Alcohol Misuse. Author:Public Health Monograph No 2; 1990.

Centers for Disease Control and Prevention (CDC). Annual smoking-attributable mortality, years of potential life lost, and economic costs – United States, 1995–9. *Morbidity and Mortality Weekly Report* 2002;51(14):300–3.

Centers for Disease Control and Prevention (CDC). Annual smoking-attributable mortality, years of potential life lost, and productivity losses – United States, 1997–2001. *Morbidity and Mortality Weekly Report* 2005;54(25):625–8.

Collins D & Lapsley, H. (May – June 2004). The social costs of smoking in Australia. *New South Wales Public Health Bulletin (15)*5–6:92–4.

Dietz VJ, Novotny TE, Rigau-Perez JG., et al. Smoking-attributable mortality, years of potential life lost, and direct health care costs for Puerto Rico, 1983. *Bulletin of PAHO* 1991;25(1):77–86.

Fenoglio P, Parel V, Kopp P. The social cost of alcohol, tobacco and illicit drugs in France, 1997. *European Addiction Research* 2003;9:18–28.

Guindon GE & Boisclair D. 2005. Costs to economy dataset 1983–2005. Prepared for the American Cancer Society; Aug 2005.

Jin S et. al. An Evaluation on Smoking-induced Health Costs in China (1988–1989). *Biomedical and Environmental Sciences* 1995;8:342–9.

Kang HY et al. Economic burden of smoking in Korea. *Tobacco Control* 2003;12(1):37–44.

McGhee SM, Hedley AJ, Ho LM. Passive smoking and its impact on employers and employees in Hong Kong. *Occupational and Environmental Medicine* 2002;59(12):842–6.

McIntyre DE, & Taylor SP.Economic aspects of smoking in South Africa. *South African Medical Journal* 1989;75(9):432–5.

Pan American Sanitary Bureau. Cost–benefit Analysis of Smoking. Caracas, Venezuela: Pan American Health Organization; 1998.

Parrott S & Godfrey C. Economic costs of smoking cessation. *BMJ* 2004;328(7445):947–9.

Pekurinen, M. (1999). *The Economic Consequences of Smoking in Finland 1987–1995*. Helsinki: Health Services Research, Ltd.

Priez F, et al. *The social cost of tobacco in Switzerland*. Institut de recherches économiques et régionales (IRER), University of Neuchâtel, Switzerland; 1999.

Rasmussen SR, Sogaard J. Socioeconomic costs due to tobacco smoking. *Ugeskr Laeger* 2000;162:3329–33.

Rath GK & Chaudry K. Cost of management of tobacco-related cancers in India. *In* Tobacco and Health (ed. K. Slama). New York: Plenum; 1995 pp. 559–564.

Sanner T. Hva koster sigarettrøykingen samfunnet? (What does cigarette smoking cost society?). *Tidsskr Nor Lægeforen* 1991;111: 3420–2.

Stephens T et al. School-based smoking cessation: economic costs versus benefits. *Chronic Diseases in Canada* 2000;21:62–7.

van Genugten MLL et al. Future burden and costs of smoking-related disease in the Netherlands: a dynamic modeling approach. *Value In Health: The Journal Of The International Society for Pharmacoeconomics and Outcomes Research* 2003;6(4):494–9.

Welte R, Konig HH, and Leidl R. Tobacco: The Costs of Health Damage and Productivity Losses Attributable to Cigarette Smoking in Germany. *European Journal of Public Health* 2000;10(1):31–8.

WHO Bangladesh. (2005). Impact of tobacco-related illnesses in Bangladesh. Document SE/BAN TOB/NCD/001 DOC/1.

Yang MC et al. Smoking attributable medical expenditures, years of potential life lost, and the cost of premature death in Taiwan. *Tobacco Control* 2005;14(Suppl 1):i62–70.

Cost of fires caused by smoking

Leistikow BN, Martin DC, Milano CE, Fire injuries, disasters, and costs from cigarettes and cigarette lights: A global overview, *Preventive Medicine* 2000;31:91.

Cost of fires caused by smoking in the USA

Federal Emergency Management Agency, US Fire Administration/National Fire Data Center, *Residential Smoking Fires and Casualties*, Topical Fire Research Series 2005:5(5). http://www.usfa.fema.gov/downloads/pdf/tfrs/v5i5.pdf Accessed Aug 2005.

Average US employee sick days per year

Halpern MT et al. Impact of smoking status on workplace absenteeism and productivity, *Tobacco Control* 2001;10:233–8.

Trash collected along the world's coasts

The Ocean Conservancy. *International Coastal Cleanup 2003*. United Kingdom Summary Report. http://www.coastalcleanup.org/documents/CountrySummaries/2003_ICC_Summary_UnitedKingdom.pdf Accessed Aug 2005.

Clipboard

Public Finance: Balance of Smoking in the Czech Republic, report commissioned by Philip Morris, Czech Republic, 2001.

Wow: USA 1997–2001

Centers for Disease Control and Prevention USA, Annual Smoking-Attributable Mortality, Years of Potential Life Lost, and Productivity Losses – United States, 1997–2001, *Morbidity and Mortality Weekly Report* 2005;54(25):625–8.

Wow: UK

Office of the Deputy Prime Minister, *Careless smoking: know the facts*, 2005. http://www.odpm.gov.uk/stellent/groups/odpm_fire/documents/page/odpm_fire_601447.hcsp. Accessed Aug 2005.

12 Costs to the smoker

Quote

Docs Fury as Reid Sparks Cigs Row Daily Record and Sunday Mail (UK), Thursday, 10 June 2004. http://www.dailyrecord.co.uk/news/tm_objectid=14318362&method=full&siteid=89488&headline=docs-fury-as-reid-sparks-cigs-row-name_page.html. Accessed Aug 2005.

Text

WHO, Tobacco Free Initiative. *Tobacco and Poverty: a vicious circle*, WHO Tobacco Control Papers; 2004.

MSN Money. The high cost of smoking. Accessed Sept 2005. http://moneycentral.msn.com/content/Insurance/Insureyourhealth/P100291.asp

The cost of smoking

White A. *A pack of Marlboros costs...* Global Partnerships for Tobacco Control, Essential Action; 2004. http://lists.essential.org/pipermail/gptc/2004q2/000130.html Accessed Aug 2005.

A hard day's smoke

Economist Intelligence Unit. Worldwide Cost of Living. March 2003 http://eiu.enumerate.com/

Union Bank of Switzerland (UBS). Prices and earnings. A comparison of purchasing power around the globe. 2003. Accessed Sept 2005. http://www.ubs.com/1/e/ubs_ch/wealth_mgmt_ch/research.html .

In 2004, for the cost of...

White A. (2004). op. cit.

Wow: Vietnam

WHO, 2004 op. cit.

PART THREE THE TOBACCO TRADE

Part-title quote

Why Iguru Will Sue Britain. All-Africa.com, 14 April 2004.

13 Growing tobacco

Text

Brown VJ. Tobacco's profit, workers' loss? *Environmental Health Perspectives* 2003;111: A284–7.

Campaign for Tobacco-Free Kids. *Global Leaf, Barren Harvest: The Costs of Tobacco Farming*. Accessed June 2005. http://tobaccofreekids.org/campaign/global/FCTCreport1.pdf.

Food and Agriculture Organization. FAOSTAT data, Tobacco Leaves: Production, 2004. http://faostat.fao.org/faostat Accessed July 2005.

Food and Agriculture Organization. FAOSTAT data, Tobacco Leaves: Area Harvested, 2004. http://faostat.fao.org/faostat Accessed July 2005.

WHO. *WHO Framework Convention on Tobacco Control, 2003*. http://www.who.int/tobacco/framework/fctc_booklet_english.pdf. Accessed June 2005.

Land devoted to growing tobacco

Food and Agriculture Organization. FAOSTAT data, Tobacco Leaves: Area Harvested, 2004 Accessed July 2005.

Food and Agriculture Organization. FAOSTAT data, Tobacco Leaves: Area Harvested, Land: Land use, Agricultural area, 2002. Accessed July 2005.

Leading producers of tobacco
Export value of tobacco
Wows

Food and Agriculture Organization. FAOSTAT data, Tobacco Leaves: Production, 2004 and 2005.

14 Cigarette manufacturing

Text

Buck D et al. *Tobacco and Jobs: The impact of reducing consumption on employment in the UK*. May 1995.

United Nations Industrial Development Organization, UNIDO INDSTAT3 2005, Industrial Statistics Database at the 3-digit level of ISIC (Rev. 2). United Nations International Standard Industrial Classification (Revision 2) at the 3-digit level: 314 Tobacco, 2005. http://www.unido.org/doc/3531.

USDA, Economic Research Service, Tobacco Statistics (94102) Table 167, World cigarette production, selected countries, 1960–95. Accessed 15 Aug 2005. http://www.ers.usda.gov/data/sdp/view.asp?f=specialty/94012

USDA, The Changing Tobacco User's Dollar, Tom Capehart: Electronic Outlook Report from the Economic Research Service, Oct 2004. Accessed 10 Aug 2005. http://www.ers.usda.gov/publications/tbs/OCT04/tbs25701 .

USDA, Tobacco and the economy: Farms, jobs and communities, Gale FH, Foreman L, and Capehart T: Agricultural Report Number 789, Economic Research Service, 2000.

Employment in cigarette factories

OECD, Structural Statistics for Industry and Services – Industrial Surveys [ISIC rev. 2] Vol 2003 release 01.

United Nations Industrial Development Organization, 2005. op. cit. (Data for Burkina Faso, Cameroon, Ghana, Australia, Portugal, Uruguay, Austria and Honduras collected from 2001 UNIDO database).

Where the tobacco dollar goes

USDA. Oct 2004 op. cit.

Less tobacco per cigarette

ERS/USDA Briefing room, Tobacco: data tables (Table 2 – Estimated leaf used for cigarettes by kind of tobacco, 1960–2003 (total domestic farm-

sales weight).
http://www.ers.usda.gov/Briefing/Tobacco/tables.
htm Accessed 15 Aug 2005.

Additives
Ingredients List: Philip Morris Web Page
http://www.philipmorrisusa.com/en/product_fa
cts/ingredients/tobacco_ingredients.asp
Accessed 15 Aug 2005.
List of Ingredients, Lorillard Tobacco Company.
Accessed 15 Aug 2005.
http://www.lorillard.com/fileadmin/user_
upload/Lorillard_Ingredients_.pdf

Wow: India
South Asian Coalition Against Child Servitude. In:
Young workers common / In India, child labor is
part of the culture by Niraj Warikoo / Free Press
Staff Writer Source: *Detroit Free Press*, 21 March
2000.

15 Tobacco companies

Text
http://www.hoovers.com/altria/--ID11179--/free-
co-factsheet.xhtml . Accessed 18 July 2005.
Altria Group, Inc. *Altria Group, Inc. 2004 Annual
Report*.
www.altria.com/investors/02_01_annualreport.a
sp . Accessed 18 July 2005.
Mackay JM. The tobacco industry in Asia:
revelations in the corporate documents. *Tobacco
Control* 2004;13 (Suppl 2): ii1–ii3.
Collin J., et al. Complicity in contraband: British
American Tobacco and cigarette smuggling in Asia.
Tobacco Control 2004;13 (Suppl 2): ii104–ii111.
Weissman R and White A. Needless Harm
International Monetary Fund Support for Tobacco
Privatization and for Tobacco Tax and Tariff
Reduction, and the Cost to Public Health: An
Essential Action Report, Sept 2002.
www.essentialaction.org/tobacco.
Lee K, Gilmore AB, Collin J. Breaking and re-
entering: British American Tobacco in China
1979–2000. *Tobacco Control* 2004;13 Suppl
2:ii88–95.
Gilmore AB et al. Pushing up smoking incidence:
plans for a privatised tobacco industry in Moldova.
Lancet 2005;365(9467):1354–9.
Philip Morris International. *Who We Are*. Accessed 18
July 2005.
www.philipmorrisinternational.com/pages/eng/o
urbus/Our_business.asp

Leading companies
ERC. *The World Cigarette Market: The 2004 Survey*.
London: ERC Group Plc; 2004
The Maxwell Report, 2004 International Tobacco Report –
Part One (April 2004), Part Two (Oct 2004), Part
One (June 2005), John C. Maxwell, Jr, 4703 Rolfe
Road Richmond, VA, 23226, USA.
The World Cigarette Guide, Tobacco Merchant's
Association, www.tma.org. Accessed 19 July
2005.

Global cigarette market share
Gallaher Group. Richard Johnson. Gallaher –
Developing Markets powerpoint presentation,
Manufacturer's reports, Euromonitor, estimates
based on ERC 2003. www.gallaher-group.com

The Big Six
Philip Morris, Net Revenues, US Securities and
Exchange Commission,
www.sec.gov/Archives/edgar/data/764180/000
095012305003146/y06457exv13.htm Accessed
22 July 2005.
JTI, *Annual report 2005*, p7, Net Sales Breakdown by
Business Segment, www.jti.co.jp Accessed 22 July
2005.
Imperial, *Annual Report 2004*, http://www.imperial-
tobacco.com Accessed 22 July 2005.
Gallaher Group, *Annual Report 2004*,
http://ir.gallaher-group.com Accessed 22 July
2005.
Altadis, *Annual Report 2004*, p. iii

JTI data for fiscal year ending March 2005. Japan
Tobacco, Inc. *Annual Report 2005*, p.62.
http://www.jti.co.jp, Accessed 19 July 2005.
Hoovers™ http://www.hoovers.com Accessed July
19, 2005.
BAT *Annual Report 2004*, www.bat.com Accessed 22
July 2005.
http://www.altadis.com Accessed 22 July 2005.

Clipboard
Where we are going…
www.bat.com/oneweb/sites/uk__3mnfen.nsf/vwP
agesWebLive/EAB16BCFCAA69CB580256BF400
0331AE?opendocument&SID=168A74A5F695F9
C50EAF26C925338773&DTC=20050718&TMP
=1) Accessed 18 July 2005.

16 Tobacco trade

Quote
Agence France Presse (AFP) (fr), 20 Aug 2004.
http://www.afp.com/quotes.php?mode=listi
ng&pattern=shigeru&records_per_page=25.
Accessed 22 Aug 2005.

Text
Food and Agriculture Organization of the United
Nations (FAO). 2005 FaoStat Statistical databases.
http://apps.fao.org

Cigarette exports
ERC. *The World Cigarette Market: The 2004 Survey*,
ERC Group Plc; 2004.
Food and Agriculture Organization of the United
Nations (FAO). 2005 FaoStat Statistical databases.
http://apps.fao.org/ [FAOSTAT code 0826].
United Nations Statistics Division. 2005 Commodity
Trade Statistics Data Base (COMTRADE).
http://esa.un.org/unsd/pubs

Top 10 leaf importers and exporters
Food and Agriculture Organization of the United
Nations (FAO). 2005 op. cit.

Tobacco leaf: US imports and exports
Cigarettes: US imports and exports
United States Department of Agriculture Foreign
Agricultural Service. *Circular Series FT-03–04*.
March 2004. Tobacco: World Markets and Trade
–Tables 6, 10, 11 and 15.

Clipboard
Tobacco Reporter, 1 Feb 2002.
http://www.tobaccoreporter.com/current/
zstory3.asp

17 Illegal cigarettes

Quote
Dr Derek Yach, Executive Director of the WHO's
Cluster on Non-Communicable Diseases and
Mental Health, 2002.
http://www.upi.com/view.cfm?StoryID=200208
01-073942-2390r

Text
Boucher P. Rendez-vous 129. Rendez-vous with Luk
Joossens. Consultant about tobacco smuggling for
WHO and UICC, Brussels, Belgium. 19 Feb
2002.
*Illegal pathways to illegal profits. The Big Cigarette
Companies and International Smuggling*. Campaign
for Tobacco-Free Kids.
http://tobaccofreekids.org/campaign/global/fra
mework/docs/Smuggling.pdf, downloaded 14 Feb
2002.
Joossens L, Raw M. Cigarette smuggling in Europe:
who really benefits? *Tobacco control* 1998;7:66–71.
Joossens L. *Technical Paper on Tobacco and Smuggling –
Questions and Answers*, Geneva: WHO, 1998.
WHO Framework Convention on Tobacco Control,
WHO; 2003.
World Bank Report, *Curbing the epidemic. Economics of
tobacco control*. Washington DC; June 1999.

Smuggled cigarettes
ERC. *The World Cigarette Market: The 2004 Survey*.
ERC Group plc; 2004.

Nguyen Thi Thanh Ha, Pham Minh Thuy, Nguyen
Song Anh, Phan Bich Khanh. *Cigarette Smuggling in
Viet Nam: Problems and Solutions*. Hanoi, 2005.

Routes:
Collin J et al. Complicity in Contraband: British
American Tobacco and Cigarette Smuggling in
Asia, *Tobacco Control* 2004:13(Suppl):ii104–ii111.
*Illegal pathways to illegal profits. The Big Cigarette
Companies and International Smuggling*. Campaign
for Tobacco-Free Kids.
http://tobaccofreekids.org/campaign/global/fra
mework/docs/Smuggling.pdf
LeGresley E. Tobacco Smuggling in Southeast Asia:
Evidence from the Industry's Documents, Penang,
Malaysia, Jan 2003.
Shafey O et al. Case Studies in international tobacco
surveillance: cigarette smuggling in Brazil. *Tobacco
Control* 2002;11:215–9.
*The cigarette "transit road" to the Islamic Republic of Iran
and Iraq: Illicit tobacco trade in the Middle East*. Cairo:
WHO EMRO; 2003.

UK seizures of smuggled cigarettes
*Measuring and Tackling Indirect Tax Losses: An Update on
the Government's Strategic Approach*, HM Customs
and Excise, HM Treasury, UK; Dec 2004 p18.
http://customs.hmrc.gov.uk/channelsPortalWeb
App/channelsPortalWebApp.portal?_nfpb=true&
_pageLabel=pageHome_ShowContent&id=HMC
E_PROD_011582&propertyType=document.

How to stop smuggling
The cigarette "transit road". op. cit

Evading duty
The World Cigarette Guide, The Tobacco Merchant's
Association 2005. http://www.tma.org

Clipboard
Cigarette Smuggling Linked to Terrorism. *The
Washington Post*, 8 June 2004.

PART FOUR PROMOTION

Part-title quote
Quoted in: EU and WHO stand shoulder to shoulder
to combat smoking,
http://europa.eu.int/comm/dgs/health_consumer
/newsletter/200202/02_en.htm

18 Marketing

Quote
Glantz SA, Kacirk KW, McCulloch C. Back to the
Future: Smoking in Movies in 2002 Compared
With 1950 Levels. *American Journal of Public Health*
2004;94:2.

Text
US Federal Trade Commission Cigarette Report for 2003,
Washington DC, USA, 2004
How Do You Sell Death. Campaign for Tobacco-Free
Kids, Washington, DC, 2001.

Leading brands
ERC. *The World Cigarette Market: The 2004 Survey*,
ERC Group Plc; 2004.
The Maxwell Report, 2004 International Tobacco Report –
Part One (April 2004) and Part Two (Oct 2004),
and Part One (June 2005), John C. Maxwell, Jr,
4703 Rolfe Road Richmond, VA, 23226, USA.
The World Cigarette Guide, The Tobacco Merchant's
Association; 2005. http://www.tma.org

Marketing expenditures
US Federal Trade Commission Cigarette Report for 2003,
Washington DC, USA; 2005.

Marketing expenditure and consumption
US Federal Trade Commission Cigarette Report for 2003.
op. cit..
Economic Research Service, USDA, Tobacco
Statistics, Table 7, Per capita consumption of
tobacco products in the United States (including
overseas forces), 1994–2004.
http://www.ers.usda.gov/briefing/tobacco/tables.
htm . Accessed 1 July 2005.

World's top-selling brands

The World Market for Tobacco, 2004
www.euromonitor.com

Honghe: The World Cigarette Guide, The Tobacco
Merchant's Association, 2005 (2005 Honghe
production volume: Jan 2005. 9B production
volume x 12 months = 108B).

The Maxwell Report, 2004. op. cit.

Top World Cigarette Market Leaders reported in
Japan Tobacco International Annual Report, p5.
Accessed 11 Aug 2005.
http://www.jti.com/english/about_jti/annual20
05_E_all.pdf .

ERC. 2004 op. cit.

Clipboard

Hamish Maxwell, PMI; 1983.
http://www.smokefreemovies.ucsf.edu/problem
/bigtobacco.html

Reynolds RJ. Tobacco Co, 1972
www.smokefreemovies.ucsf.edu

Silver screen

Glantz SA, Kacirk KW, McCulloch C. 2004 op. cit.

19 Buying influence

Quote

Common Cause President, Chellie Pingree, 2004
http://tobaccofreekids.org/Script/DisplayPressR
elease.php3?Display=791

Knight J and Chapman S. "A phoney way to show
sincerity, as we all well know": tobacco industry
lobbying against tobacco control in Hong Kong.
Tobacco Control 2004;13(Supp II):ii13–ii21.

Text

Tobacco-Free Kids and Common Cause (2004).
*Campaign Contributions By Tobacco Interests; Annual
Report: October 2004.* Available at
http://tobaccofreeaction.org

Hammond R and Rowell A *Trust Us: We're the Tobacco
Industry.* Campaign for Tobacco-Free Kids. (2001).
Accessed July 20, 2005.
http://www.ash.org.uk/html/conduct/html/trus
tus.html#_Toc514752794

Tobacco Industry Gave Nearly $2.8 Million in
Federal Political Contributions So Far in the
2003–4 Election Cycle: Members Who Voted
Against FDA Tobacco Regulation Got Five Times
as Much Tobacco Money, 21 Oct 2004
http://tobaccofreekids.org/Script/DisplayPressR
elease.php3?Display=791

Clipboards on map

Small shopkeepers…
Philip Morris 10 Aug 1990. Industry response to,
and impact of, anti-tobacco legislation in Canada.
From Landman Collection 2026230531-0540.

We have got the unions….
Philip Morris: The Perspective of PM International
on Smoking and Health Issues, 27 March 1985.
Quoted in Landman's Collection
landman/2023268351-8364:7.

Philip Morris and the Industry
Philip Morris Corporate Affairs Plan. 25 Nov 1987.
From Landman collection 2501254715-4723.

Turning now…
Philip Morris. 1985 op. cit.

Mongoven J. 19971100. Philip Morris and analysis of
WHO convention (FCTC) process. Access Date:
July 14, 2005. Bates No: 2074292078/2082.
http://www.pmdocs.com/getallimg.asp?if=avpid
x&DOCID=2074292078/2082

Unless countervailing…
Reynolds RJ. document, 1978, Landman Collection,
Bates No. 500851221-500851262.

What are we trying to accomplish…
Document Type: Report, Date: 03/20/1990,
Author: N/A, Title: Top Secret Operation
Rainmaker, Site: Philip Morris document site,
Bates No. 2048302227/2230.
http://www.pmdocs.com/getallimg.asp?DOCID
=2048302227/2230

Buying influence
Buying favours

Tobacco-Free Kids and Common Cause (2004).
*Campaign Contributions By Tobacco Interests; Annual
Report: October 2004.* Available at
http://tobaccofreeaction.org

20 Tobacco industry documents

Text

British American Tobacco Document Collection,
Digital Library of University of California, San
Francisco.
http://www.library.ucsf.edu/tobacco/batco

Framework Convention Alliance for Tobacco
Control, Tobacco Industry Documents – Factsheet
No 6, 2005.
http://www.fctc.org/factsheets/index.php
Accessed 15 Aug 2005.

Glantz SA, Slade J, Bero LA, Hanauer P, Barnes DE
(eds), *The Cigarette Papers,* University of California
Press, 1996.

Legacy Foundation site,
http://legacy.library.ucsf.edu/ Accessed 15 Aug
2005.

Legacy website

Authors search using country names, Legacy
Foundation site, http://legacy.library.ucsf.edu
August 2005.

Clipboards

Our work in Senegal…
A law prohibiting
Whist A Philip Morris Memorandum. 17 Dec 1986.
Bates No. 2025431401/1406.
http://www.pmdocs.com/getallimg.asp?DOCID
=2025431401/1406.

Work to develop…
Philip Morris, 1987, as quoted in *Voices of Truth,* Vol 2.

Asia is now…
Dollisson J. Philip Morris 2nd Revised Forecast
Presentation. June 1989 (est)
Bates No. 2500101311/1323.
http://www.pmdocs.com/getallimg.asp?if=avpidx&
DOCID=2500101311/1323.

Naturally…
Kornegay H. Tobacco Institute, Speech to Tobacco
and Allied Industries Division of the American
Jewish Community on Dec 11, 1979. Bates No.
TIMN0094652-4662.
http://www.tobaccodocuments.org/view.cfm?do
cid=TIMN0094652/4662&source=SNAPTI&Sho
wImages=yes

Document retention policy
Kremner C. US seeks facts on smoke conspiracy. *The
Age.* 19 April 2002
http://www.theage.com.au/articles/2002/04/18/
1019020683796.html

Wow: nearly 300 research reports

Norbert Hirschhorn MD, Research Reports and
Publications Based on Tobacco Industry
Documents, 1991–2005, May 2005, 7th edition

PART FIVE TAKING ACTION

21 Research

Quote

Lando HA, Borrelli B, Klein LC, Waverly LP,
Stillman FA, Kassel JD, Warner KE. The
Landscape in Global Tobacco Control Research: A
Guide to Gaining a Foothold. *American Journal of
Public Health* 2005;95(6): 939–45.

Text

Baris et al., Research priorities for tobacco control
in developing countries: A regional approach to a
global consultative process. *Tobacco Control* 9:
217–23, 2000.

Bero LA, Glantz S, Hong M-K. The limits of
competing interest disclosures. *Tobacco Control*
2005;14:118–26.

Tobacco control research projects

Community Actions to Prevent Chronic Diseases
(CAPCoD) projects sponsored by the Oxford
Health Alliance: Personal communication,
Professor Derek Yach, Yale School of Public
Health, 24 May 2005.

Fogarty:
http://www.fic.nih.gov/news/newsletter/Aug20
03/map.htm
http://www.fic.nih.gov/programs/tobacco.html
Accessed 2 May 2005.

Global Youth Tobacco Survey, Countries that have
and are implementing or planning to complete
survey in 2004
http://www.cdc.gov/tobacco/global/GYTS.htm

IDRC: Personal communication, Rosemary
Kennedy, RITC Research Officer and Coordinator,
April 20, 2005,
http://archive.idrc.ca/ritc/en/projects/index.html

Institute for Global Tobacco Control/GTRN:
Personal communication, Carrie Mattson, IGTC
Senior Research Program Coordinator, 18 May
2005.

ITEN – International Tobacco Evidence Network
Personal communication, Han Ross, RTI
International Research Economist, 23 April 2005,
http://www.tobaccoevidence.net

Rockefeller Foundation:
http://www.lshtm.ac.uk/cgch/tobacco/rockefell
er_project.htm and Lando HA, Borrelli B et al.
The Landscape in Global Tobacco Control
Research: A Guide to Gaining a Foothold.
American Journal of Public Health 2005;95(6):
939–45.

Swedish International Development Cooperation
Agency (Sida): Lando HA et al. The Landscape in
Global Tobacco Control Research: A Guide to
Gaining a Foothold. *American Journal of Public
Health* 2005;95(6):939–45.

UNF: http://www.who.int/tobacco/research/youth/
alliances/en/
http://w3.whosea.org/rdhome/rdreport02/ch2.
htm, "Channel the Outrage"
http://w3.whosea.org/EN/Section1174/section
1462/TFIMain.asp?pg=ngolist2
http://www.who.int/tobacco/training/projects/en/,
accessed 2 May 2005.

How much research?

US National Library of Medicine, PubMed search, 3
March 2005.

Comparative research expenditure

Data derived from Research expenditures are from
the US National Institutes of Health estimates for
2003. The deaths are preliminary for 2003 and the
source is Table 2 of *National Vital Statistics Report*
2005:53(15).

Flegal, Katherine M. et al., Excess Deaths Associated
with Underweight, Overweight and Obesity.
JAMA 2005;293(15).

http://www.cdc.gov/cvh/library/fs_stroke.htm,
accessed 25 April 2005.

http://www.cdc.gov/tobacco/factsheets/Tobacco_
Related_Mortality_factsheet.htm . Accessed 25
April 2005.

Smoking-Attributable Mortality (United States,
2001) SAMMEC,
http://apps.nccd.cdc.gov/sammec/sam_reports.
asp . Accessed 6 May 2005.

22 Capacity building

Quote

World Tobacco Free Initiative, Building blocks for
tobacco control: a handbook, pxiii, available
online, p. xIII.
http://www.who.int/tobacco/resources/publicat
ions/general/HANDBOOK%20Lowres%20with
%20cover.pdf Accessed 27 July 2005.

Text

Stillman F et al. Building Capacity for International
Tobacco Control Research: The Global Tobacco

Research Network. *American Journal of Public Health* 2005;95(6):965–8.

Wipfli H, Stillman F, Tamplin S, Luiza da Costa e Silva V, Yack D, Samet J. Achieving the Framework Convention on Tobacco Control's potential by investing in national capacity. *Tobacco Control* 2004;13:433–7.

World Tobacco Free Initiative, *Building blocks for tobacco control: a handbook*. http://www.who.int/tobacco/resources/publications/general/HANDBOOK%20Lowres%20with%20cover.pdf Accessed 27 July 2005.

Plans of action
11th WCTOH, Personal Communication, Omar Shafey, ACS, 15 July 2005.

ACS/UICC, Tobacco Control Research, ACS/UICC/CRUK, Tobacco Control Research, ACS/CRTCI/RITC, Tobacco Control Research, Romania Tobacco Seed Grants, Tobacco Control research,
http://www.cancer.org/docroot/AA/content/AA_2_5_5x_Tobacco_Control_Research.asp?sitearea=AA. Accessed 20 July 2005.

Pacific Island States, Personal Communication, Rosemary Kennedy, Research Officer and Coordinator, RITC, 24 May 2005. http://archive.idrc.ca/ritc/en/activities/strengthening2.html

WHO Capacity Building, Global Projects, TFI Seed Grants and other projects
http://www.who.int/tobacco/training/global_projects/en/index.html. Accessed 20 July 2005.
http://www.who.int/tobacco/training/projects/en/index.html. Accessed 20 July 2005.

WHO: Other projects for strengthening national capacity.
http://www.who.int/tobacco/training/projects/en/index.html. Accessed 29 July 2005.

Key strategies to strengthen national capacity for tobacco control
WHO
http://www.who.int/tobacco/training/strategies/en/index.html Accessed 20 July 2005.

Additional organizations
Personal communication, Laurent Huber at Framework Convention Alliance for Tobacco Control, www.fctc.org, 9 Sept 2005.

Norwegian Cancer Society, Personal Communication, Bjarne Rosted, Senior Adviser International Affairs, NCS, 5 Aug 2005.

23 FCTC

Signatories to WHO FCTC
http://www.who.int/en Accessed 1 Dec 2004.

Support for WHO FCTC
Public Support for International Efforts to Control Tobacco: A Survey in Five Countries. PN4808. Draft Report (2). Prepared for WHO by Environics Research Group Ltd. 27 April 2001.

24 Smoke-free areas

Quote
Americans for Nonsmokers' Rights, *Ventilation and Air Filtration: What Air Filtration Companies and the Tobacco Industry Are Saying.* http://www.no-smoke.org/document.php?id=267. Accessed July 2005.

Text
Americans for Nonsmokers' Rights, Patron surveys and consumer behavior. http://www.no-smoke.org/pdf/patronsurveys.pdf Accessed July 2005.

Quinet M, Orban M, Philippet C, Riffon A, Andrien M. *Non-smokers protection in restaurants and bars in Europe: A survey in five European countries, European Network for Smoking Prevention.* Europe Against Cancer.
http://www.fares.be/tabagisme/news/surveyHo

recaFinalReport.pdf Accessed June 2005.

Raaijmakers T, van den Borne I, Cost-benefits of workplace smoking policies. In: *Smoke free workplaces: improving the health and well-being of people at work, European Status Report.* 2001. Fleitman S (ed). European Network for Smoking Prevention. http://www.ensp.org/reports.cfm. Accessed July 2005.

Smoke-free areas at work
ASH Scotland, ASH Scotland Briefing, Smoke-free Legislation around the World. http://www.ashscotland.org.uk/ash/files/ASH%20Scotland%20Smoke%20Free%20Legislation%20around%20the%20World%20Briefing%202.doc Accessed June 2005.

ERC Group plc, World Cigarettes 2, The 2004 Survey. Health Legislation Unit, WHO, International Digest of Health Legislation. http://www3.who.int/idhl-rils/frame.cfm?language=english Accessed June 2005.

Ireland: http://data.euro.who.int/tobacco/Default.aspx?TabID=2404

National Tobacco Information Online System (NATIONS). http://apps.nccd.cdc.gov/nations/ Accessed June 2005.

Shafey O, Dolwick S, Guindon GE (eds). *Tobacco Control Country Profiles 2003*, American Cancer Society, Atlanta, GA, 2003.

WHO EMRO, Tobacco Free Initiative. *Country Profiles on Tobacco Control in the Eastern Mediterranean Region.* http://www.emro.who.int/tfi/country profile.htm Accessed June 2005.

WHO EURO, Tobacco Free Initiative, Tobacco control database. http://data.euro.who.int/tobacco/ Accessed June 2005.

WHO SEARO, Tobacco Free Initiative, Country Data on Tobacco Control. http://tfi.wpro.who.int/country_specific_indicators.asp Accessed June 2005.

WHO SEARO, Tobacco Free Initiative, Legislative measures in SEAR Countries. http://w3.whosea.org/EN/Section1174/section1462/TFIMain.asp?pg=legislative Accessed June 2005.

Costs of workplace smoking
Griffiths J, Grieves K. *Why Smoking in the Workplace Matters: An Employers Guide.* WHO European Partnership Project to Reduce Tobacco Dependence, 2002:3.

Polluted air in hospitals
Navas-Acien A et al. Secondhand tobacco smoke in public places in Latin America, 2002–3, *Journal of the American Medical Association* 2004;291(22):2741–5.

Navas-Acien A, Peruga A, personal communication, 24 June 2005.

Nebot M, et al, Environmental tobacco smoke exposure in public places of European cities, *Tobacco Control* 2005;14(1):60–3.

No loss of restaurant and bar sales
California Board of Equalization, 1997,1998, 1999, 2000, 2001, 2002, 2003, 2004 http://www.boe.ca.gov/news Accessed July 2005.

California Department of Health, California Board of Equalization, Before and After Smoke-free Laws First Quarter Taxable Sales Figures for Restaurants & Bars, State of California 1992–9. In: Repace J. *Can Ventilation Control Secondhand Smoke in the Hospitality Industry?* June 2000. Figure 3:34. http://www.repace.com

Clipboard
Hieronimus J, *Memorandum: Impact of workplace restrictions on consumption and incidence*, Philip Morris, USA, 22 October 1992, Bates No.: 2023914280/4284
http://www.pmdocs.com/getallimg.asp?if=avpidx&DOCID=2023914280/4284 Accessed July 2005.

25 Marketing restrictions

Quote
Lewis S. http://www.quotationspage.com/quote/841.html. Accessed July, 2005.

Text
Assunta M, Chapman S. "The world's most hostile environment": how the tobacco industry circumvented Singapore's advertising ban. *Tobacco Control* 2004;13 Suppl 2:ii51–7.

Assunta M, Chapman S. The tobacco industry's accounts of refining indirect tobacco advertising in Malaysia. *Tobacco Control* 2004;13 Suppl 2:ii63–70.

Carter SM. New frontier, new power: the retail environment in Australia's dark market. *Tobacco Control* 2003;12 Suppl 3:iii95–101.

Saffer H, Chaloupka F, The effect of tobacco advertising bans on tobacco consumption. *Journal of Health Economics* 2000;19:1117–37.

The World Bank. *Curbing the Epidemic: Governments and the Economics of Tobacco Control.* The World Bank, Washington DC, USA; 1999.

Wakefield M et al, The cigarette pack as image: new evidence from tobacco industry documents, *Tobacco Control* 2002;11 Suppl 1:i73–80.

Wakefield M, Letcher T, My pack is cuter than your pack, *Tobacco Control* 2002;11:154–6.

Media bans
ASH Scotland, *ASH Scotland Briefing. Smoke-free Legislation around the World.* Accessed June, 2005. http://www.ashscotland.org.uk/ash/files/ASH%20Scotland%20Smoke%20Free%20Legislation%20around%20the%20World%20Briefing%202.doc

ERC Group plc. *World Cigarettes 2, The 2004 Survey,* Suffolk, UK.

Health Legislation Unit, WHO, *International Digest of Health Legislation.* http://www3.who.int/idhl-rils/frame.cfm?language=english Accessed June, 2005.

National Tobacco Information Online System (NATIONS), http://apps.nccd.cdc.gov/nations/ Accessed June, 2005.

Shafey O, Dolwick S, Guindon GE (eds), *Tobacco Control Country Profiles 2003,* American Cancer Society, Atlanta, GA, USA; 2003.

WHO EMRO, Tobacco Free Initiative, *Country Profiles on Tobacco Control in the Eastern Mediterranean Region.* http://www.emro.who.int/tfi/country profile.htm Accessed June 2005.

WHO EURO. Tobacco Free Initiative. *Tobacco control database.* http://data.euro.who.int/tobacco/ Accessed June, 2005.

WHO SEARO, Tobacco Free Initiative, *Country Data on Tobacco Control.* http://tfi.wpro.who.int/country_specific_indicators.asp Accessed June, 2005.

WHO SEARO, Tobacco Free Initiative, *Legislative measures in SEAR Countries.* http://w3.whosea.org/EN/Section1174/section1462/TFIMain.asp?pg=legislative Accessed June, 2005.

Brand stretching
Global Youth Tobacco Survey Collaborating Group. *Global Youth Tobacco Survey Country Fact Sheets.* Centers for Disease Control and Prevention. http://www.cdc.gov/tobacco/Global/gyts/GYTS_factsheets.htm Accessed June 2005.

Clipboard
Miller L, *Principles of measurement of visual standout in pack design, Report No. 2039 Restricted,* Group Research & Development Centre, British American Tobacco Co. Ltd., May 23 1986, Bates No. 102699347-102699500.

Wow: Singapore
WHO, *Tobacco or health: a global status report.* 1997:482–5.

Wow: comprehensive advertising bans
Saffer H, Chaloupka F. The effect of tobacco advertising bans on tobacco consumption. *Journal of Health Economics* 2000;19:1117–37.

26 Warning labels

Quote

ASH Scotland. *Policy Paper on Regulation and Control of Tobacco Products: Packaging/Labelling.* Accessed April 2002 (no longer available). http://www.ashsscotland.org.uk/issues/tob_reg09.html

Text

Campaign for Tobacco-Free Kids. *Tobacco Warning Labels and Packaging Fact Sheet.* 11th World Conference on Tobacco or Health; 2000. http://tobaccofreekids.org/campaign/global/docs/warning.pdf Accessed June 2005.

Cavalcante TM, *Labelling and packaging in Brazil,* WHO; 2003. http://www.who.int/tobacco/training/success_stories/en/best_practices_brazil_labelling.pdf Accessed June 2005.

Cunningham R. *Package Warnings: Overview of International Developments.* Canadian Cancer Society; 2004.

GLOBALink. *UICC Tobacco Control Fact Sheet 2: Health warnings/messages on tobacco products* Accessed June 2005.http://www.globalink.org/tobacco/fact_sheets/02fact.htm

WHO. *Framework Convention on Tobacco Control.* Geneva: WHO/TFI. http://www.who.int/tobacco/framework/fctc_booklet_english.pdf Accessed June 2005.

Health warnings on packs of cigarettes
Health warnings on tobacco advertisements

ASH Scotland. ASH Scotland Briefing. *Smoke-free Legislation around the World.* http://www.ashsscotland.org.uk/ash/files/ASH%20Scotland%20Smoke%20Free%20Legislation%20around%20the%20World%20Briefing%202.doc Accessed June 2005.

ERC Group plc. *World Cigarette Report 2, The 2004 Survey.*

Health Legislation Unit. WHO. *International Digest of Health Legislation.* http://www3.who.int/idhl-rils/frame.cfm?language=english Accessed June 2005.

National Tobacco Information Online System (NATIONS). http://apps.nccd.cdc.gov/nations Accessed June 2005.

Shafey O, Dolwick S, Guindon GE (eds). *Tobacco Control Country Profiles 2003.* American Cancer Society. Atlanta, GA; 2003.

WHO EMRO. Tobacco Free Initiative. *Country Profiles on Tobacco Control in the Eastern Mediterranean Region.* http://www.emro.who.int/tfi/countryprofile.htm Accessed June 2005.

WHO EURO. Tobacco Free Initiative, *Tobacco control database.* http://data.euro.who.int/tobacco Accessed June 2005.

WHO SEARO. Tobacco Free Initiative. *Country Data on Tobacco Control.* http://tfi.wpro.who.int/country_specific_indicators.asp Accessed June 2005.

WHO SEARO. Tobacco Free Initiative. *Legislative measures in SEAR Countries.* http://w3.whosea.org/EN/Section1174/section1462/TFIMain.asp?pg=legislative Accessed June 2005.

Clipboard

Chapman S, Carter SM. "Avoid health warnings on all tobacco products for just as long as we can": a history of Australian tobacco industry efforts to avoid, delay and dilute health warnings on cigarettes. *Tobacco Control* 2003;12: Suppl 3:iii13–22.

Influence of cigarette pack labels
Wow: Canada

Fong G. Personal communication, 10 June 2005.

27 Health education

Quote

Peterson Jr. AV et al. Hutchinson Smoking Prevention Project: Long-Term Randomized trial in School-Based Tobacco use Prevention – Results on Smoking. *Journal of the National Cancer Institute* 2000;92(24):1988.

Text

British American Tobacco Accessed 29 April 2005.<http://www.bat.com/oneweb/sites/uk_3mnfen.nsf/vwPagesWebLive/00EE816257C9ACD480256BF4000331D7?opendocument&SID=7908A0FF587E5A58D163339763AB6170&DTC=20050429&TMP=1

Phillip Morris International Accessed 29 April 2005. http://www.altria.com/about_altria/01_05_04_pmistory.asp & http://www.altria.com/about_altria/01_00_02_PhilipMorrisIntl.asp

Quit & Win campaign

Personal communication. Marjo Pyykönen. Coordinator, International Quit&Win. 25 April 2005

Annual themes of World No Tobacco Day

WHO http://www.who.int/tobacco/communications/events/wntd/en/

Clipboard

Discussion Paper. 29 Jan 1991. Site: Tobacco Institute document site http://tobaccoinstitute.com/ Bates No. TIMN0164422/4424 (and also other Bates No. TIFL0526381/6383) http://www.tobaccoinstitute.com/getallimg.asp?DOCID=TIMN0164422/4424

28 Quitting

Quote

Thomas Carlyle, Scottish writer and journalist (1795–1881). http://www.motivatingquotes.com/healthq.htm Accessed 29 April 2005.

Ex-smokers

Personal communication (JM). World Self-Medication Industry. April 2002.
World Self Medication Industry. OTC Ingredients, Non-Prescription Ingredients Classification Tables. 2004. http://www.wsmi.org/otc.htm Accessed 8 Aug 2005.

Algeria – 2000. 11th World Conference on Tobacco or Health: Abstracts Vol.2 (Chicago, IL).
Austria –*Wiener Medizinische Wochenschrift* 2000;150(6):109–114.
Bahamas –*Tobacco or Health: Status in the Americas* 1992. Washington DC.
Chile –*Pan American Journal of Public Health* 2000;7(2):79–87.
China –*Tobacco Control* 2001;10(2):170–4.
Côte d'Ivoire – *Poumon-Coeur.* 1981.37:87–94.
Cyprus – Research Papers and Reports: Series II. Report no. 19. ISBN 9963-34-344-9.
Czech Republic – *Casopis Lekaru Ceskych* 2000;139(5):143–147.
Denmark – *International Journal of Epidemiology* 1992;21(5):862–71.
Dominican Republic –*Bulletin of PAHO* 1993;27(4):370–381.
Ecuador – *see* Bahamas.
Egypt –Provided to the ACS; from the first cycle of The Health Interview Survey of Egypt; 1982.
Finland –Provided to the ACS; data from Health Behavior among Finnish Adult Population – spring 1998.
France –*International Journal of Tuberculosis and Lung Disease* 2000;4(8):698–704.
Germany – *Jahrbuch Sucht* 1999.
Ghana – a pamphlet sent to ACS by the Health and Humanitarian Environment Society.
Honduras – *see* Bahamas.

Iran (Islamic Republic of) — *see* Algeria.
Israel –*The Israeli Medical Journal* 2000;2(5):351–5.
Kuwait – *Bulletin of the WHO* 2000;78(11):1306–1315.
Malawi – *Tropical Doctor* 1996;26(3),139.
Mexico – Unpublished Data; 1998.
Peru – PAHO publication; 1992.
Russian Federation – *see* Algeria.
Saudi Arabia – National Study on Coronary Artery Risk Factors; 1996–2001.
South Africa – *see* Algeria.
Sudan – *see* Algeria.
Sweden – *Tobacco Control* 2001;10:258–266.
Thailand – 1993. Thailand's Situation. Online: www.ash.or.th/situation/women.htm
Tonga – *Tobacco Control* 1994;3:41–45.
Trinidad and Tobago — *see* Bahamas.
Tuvalu – *Bulletin of the WHO* 1986;64(3):447–456, data was provided to the ACS.
USA – *see* Bahamas.
Uruguay – *see* Bahamas.
Venezuela – 1994, provided to the ACS via fax.
Zambia – pre-publication results of a survey in Mutendere, a suburb of Lusaka. Mulenga M, Haworth A, Mwanza P.

Effects of starting and quitting smoking on deaths

Peto R, Lopez AD. The future worldwide health effects of current smoking patterns. In: Koop EC, Pearson CE, Schwarz MR, eds. *Critical Issues in Global Health.* New York: Jossey-Bass; 2001:154–61.

Why people give up smoking

Public Health Statistics on NHS Stop Smoking Services, p21. http://www.dh.gov.uk/PublicationsAndStatistics/Statistics/StatisticalWorkAreas/StatisticalPublicHealth/fs/en. Accessed 27 July 2005.

Effectiveness of workplace smoking cessation programmes

Smedslund G et al. The effectiveness of workplace smoking cessation programmes: a meta-analysis of recent studies. *Tobacco Control* 2004;13:197–204.

Clipboard

Smoking and Health Vol I Fourth Edition 760700 A Documentation for PME Personnel Type of Document: Report Author: Gaisch H. and Gustafson B. (Philip Morris Europe) Date: 19760700 Page Count: 58 Site: Philip Morris Document site http://www.pmdocs.com/cgi-bin/rsasearch.exe #1 Bates No. 1002635107/5164.

Wow: USA

World Self-Medication Industry. About self-medication: Society and public health. http://www.wsmi.org/aboutsm1.htm Accessed 9 Aug 2005.

29 Tobacco taxes

Quote

Smith A. *An Inquiry into the Nature and Causes of the Wealth of Nations.* London: Methuen & Co Ltd, 1776.

Text

Jha P and Chaloupka F. *Tobacco Control in Developing Countries.* Oxford: Oxford University Press; 2000.
Jha P and Chaloupka F. *Curbing the Epidemic: Governments and the Economics of Tobacco Control.* Washington DC: World Bank; 1999.

Tax as a proportion of cigarette price

Guindon GE & Boisclair D. Tobacco Taxation dataset 1999–2005. Prepared for the American Cancer Society, Aug 2005.
Perucic AM. Tobacco Tax Earmarking dataset. Prepared for the American Cancer Society; Aug 2005.

Smoking goes down as prices go up

Van Walbeek C. *Tobacco Excise Taxation in South Africa.*

Geneva: WHO; 2003.

Government income from tobacco
Guindon GE, Perucic AM, Boisclair D. *Higher Tobacco Prices and Taxes in South East Asia: An Effective Tool to Reduce Tobacco Use, Save Lives and Generate Revenue.* Tobacco Control: WHO Tobacco Control Papers. Paper SEASIA2003. 2003. http://repositories.cdlib.org/tc/whotcp/SEASIA 2003. Accessed Sept 2004.

Tax down – but prices up
Orzechowski W and Walker RC. Tax Burden on Tobacco. Arlington, Virginia: Orzechowski and Walker; 2004.

Clipboard
Walls T. "Grasstops Government Relations." Philip Morris. Bates number 2024023252/3265. 30 March 1993. http://www.pmdocs.com Accessed Sept 2005.

Wow: China
Hu TW and Mao Z. Effects of cigarette tax on cigarette consumption and the Chinese economy. *Tobacco Control* 2002;11(2):105–8.

30 Litigation
Quote
Personal communication with Professor Richard Daynard, Professor of Law, Northeastern University, USA; 2005.

Text
Blanke DD. Towards Health with Justice: Litigation and public inquiries as tools for tobacco control, WHO; 18 March 2002 http://tobacco.who.int/repository/stp69/final_jordan_report.pdf ID:88634.
Walburn RB. The prospects for globalizing tobacco litigation, WHO's International Conference on Global Tobacco Control Law: Towards a WHO Framework Convention on Tobacco Control, New Delhi, India; 7 Jan 2000.

Lawsuits
Altadis Annual Report 2004. Litigation. p25. http://www.altadis.com/en/shareholders/pdf/meeting2005/infoanual2004.pdf
Altria Group Annual Report 2004. Overview of Tobacco-Related Litigation. p.67. http://www.altria.com/AnnualReport/ar2004 Accesssed 20 July 2005.
BAT Annual Report 2004. US and Other Foreign Litigation, pp27–8. http://www.bat.com Accessed 20 July 2005.
Gallaher Annual Report 2004. Legal and Regulatory Environment. http://ir.gallaher-group.com/ir/publications/2004_report/legal_and_reg.asp Accessed 20 July 2005.
Imperial Tobacco Annual Report 2004, Operating Environment: Tobacco Related Litigation. http://www.imperialtobacco.com/prelim_results_2004/sites/?pageid=47
JTI Annual Report 2004. Tobacco-related Litigation. pp51–3. http://www.jti.com/english/about_jti/annual2005_E_all.pdf Accessed 20 July 2005.

A range of lawsuits
Rising anti-tobacco litigation
Altria Group, Inc. *Altria Group, Inc. 2004 Annual Report.* Accessed 20 July 2005. http://www.altria.com/investors/02_01_annualreport.asp, p67.
Altria Group, Inc. Form 10-Q. U.S. Securities and Exchange Commission. submitted 5 Aug 2005.

Clipboard
Edwards J. Report from Philip Morris Counsel to Philip Morris Counsel Regarding Meeting on Addiction. 6 Nov 1986. Bates No.:2025005346/5367, http://www.tobaccodocuments.org/view.cfm?docid=25156&source=BLILEY&ShowImages=yes

Wow: USA – BAT
BAT Annual Report 2004. Annual Review and Summary Financial Statement 2004. US Litigation. pp27–8. http://www.bat.com Accessed 20 July 2005.

Wow: USA – Philip Morris
Janofsky Michael. Big Tobacco, in Court Again. But the Stock Is Still Up. *New York Times.* 14 Aug 2005. http://www.nytimes.com/2005/08/14/politics/14tobacco.html?ex=1124596800&en=b859ba06847779ab&ei=5070&emc=eta1

31 The future
Mackay J. Lessons from the Conference: The Next 25 Years.10th World Conference on Tobacco or Health. Beijing, China; 24–28 Aug 1997.
Future Scenarios Plenary: Tobacco Control 2015: Where, Why and With What Outcomes? 11th World Conference on Tobacco or Health. Chicago Illinois; 6–11 Aug 2000.

Number of smokers
Personal communication. WHO/EIP via Emmanuel Guindon; 3 June 2002.
WHO. *Why is tobacco a public health priority?* http://www.who.int/tobacco/en Accessed 05 May 2005.

Health
WHO. *Why is tobacco a public health priority?* ibid.
WHO. The World Health Report 2002: reducing risks, promoting healthy life. Geneva: WHO; 2002:65.
Personal communication, Alan Lopez. 12 April 2002. From Lopez and Peto 2001.

32 The history of tobacco
Borio G. Tobacco Timeline. Accessed 27 July. 2005.http://www.tobacco.org/resources/history/Tobacco_History18.html
Cochran S. Big Business in China: Sino–Foreign Rivalry in the Cigarette Industry, 1890–1930. Harvard University Press; 1980.
Framingham Heart Study. A Timeline of Milestones. http://www.framingham.com/heart/timeline.htm
Globalink. Tobaccopedia. http://tobaccopedia.org/cgi-local/seek.cgi. Accessed 16 July 2005.
Jelbert H. *Tobacco – A brief history.* Health Education Authority, UK.
Kluger R. *Ashes to Ashes: America's Hundred-Year War, the Public Health and the Unabashed Triumph of Philip Morris.* Alfred A Knopf, New York; 1996.
Hong-Gwan Seo. Chairman of Smoking Cessation Clinic, National Cancer Center, Republic of Korea. Personal communication. 1 Aug 2005.
Lyons AS, Petrucelli RJ II. *Medicine: An illustrated history.* Harry N Abrams Inc, New York; 1978:580.
Moyer D. *The Tobacco Almanac: A reference book of fact, figures, quotations about tobacco.* David B. Moyer, Navy Surgeon General's expert on tobacco; Oct 1998 (self published).
Routh HB, Bhowmik KR, Parish JL, Parish LC. Historical Aspects of Tobacco Use and Smoking. *Clinics in Dermatology* 1998;16(5):539–544.
The Faber Book of Smoking, 2000.
Tobacco milestones: A brief history of tobacco. adapted from a chronology by the National Clearinghouse on Tobacco and Health, Ottawa, Canada; 1996.
Tobacco Facts. Tobacco Truth: From first drag to slavery: tobacco's beginnings. http://www.tobaccofacts.org/tob_truth/timeline1492.html. Accessed 10 Oct 2004.

PART SIX TABLES

Part-title quote
http://www.tobacco.org/quotes.php?mode=listing&pattern=omi&records_per_page=25

Table A The demographics of tobacco
1 Population
http://www.who.int
UN Population and Vital Statistics Report: Series A, Table 2. Population, latest available census and estimates for 2002 or 2003. http://unstats.un.org/unsd/demographic/products/vitstats/seriesa2.htm Accessed 30 Sept 2005.
2 Adult smoking prevalence
See sources above for **2 Male smoking, Smoking prevalence for men**
3 Health professionals' smoking prevalence
See sources above for **4 Health professionals, Smoking prevalence among health professionals**
4 Youth smoking prevalence
See sources above for **5 Boys' tobacco use, Early starters**
5 Passive smoking
See sources above for **9 Passive smoking, Domestic danger**
6 Cigarette consumption
See sources above for **7 Cigarette consumption, Annual cigarette consumption.**

Table B The business of tobacco
1 Growing tobacco
Columns 1 & 2: *see sources above for* **13 Growing tobacco, Land devoted to growing tobacco**
column 3: *see sources above for* **13 Growing tobacco, Leading producers of tobacco.**
2 Tobacco trade
columns 1 & 2: *see sources above for* **16 Tobacco trade, Cigarette exports**
columns 3 & 4: *see sources above for* **16 Tobacco trade, Top 10 leaf exporters/importers**
3 Manufacturing
column 1: *See sources above for* **14 Cigarette manufacturing, Employment in cigarette factories**
column 2: ERC. *The World Cigarette Market: The 2004 Survey.* London: ERC Group Plc; 2004
United Nations Statistics Division. Industrial Commodities Production Yearbook and Database. 2005. http://unstats.un.org/unsd/cdb/cdb_series_xrx.asp?series_code=18090
United States Department of Agriculture Foreign Agricultural Service Tobacco: World Markets and Trade Special Report – World Cigarette Tables, Circular Series FT-09-04 Sept 2004. http://www.fas.usda.gov/tobacco/circular/2004/092004/indexSep.htm
4 Price
column 1: *see sources above for* **12 Costs to the smoker, The cost of smoking**
5 Tax
See sources above for **29 Tobacco taxes, Tax as a proportion of cigarette price**
6 WHO FCTC
columns 1 & 2: *see sources above for* **23 Framework Convention on Tobacco Control, Signatories to FCTC**
7 Tobacco industry documents
see sources above for **20 Tobacco industry documents, Legacy website.**

USEFUL CONTACTS

Online edition of this atlas: Global Tobacco Research Network
http://www.tobaccoresearch.net/atlas.html

WHO Tobacco Free Initiative

WHO Headquarters
  http://tobacco.who.int/
AFRO
  http://www.whoafr.org/tfi/index.html
EMRO
  http://www.emro.who.int/tfi/tfi.htm
EURO
  http://www.who.dk/eprise/main/WHO/Progs/TOB/Home
PAHO
  http://www.paho.org/
SEARO
  http://w3.whosea.org/techinfo/index.htm
WPRO
  http://www.wpro.who.int/themes_focuses/theme2/special/tobacco.asp

International Organizations

Action on Smoking and Health
  http://www.ash.org.uk/
British American Tobacco Document Collection
  http://www.library.ucsf.edu/tobacco/batco/
Campaign for Tobacco Free Kids
  http://www.tobaccofreekids.org/
Framework Convention Alliance for Tobacco Control (FCA)
  http://www.fctc.org/
FCTCnow!
  http://www.fctcnow.org
Global Partnerships for Tobacco Control
  http://www.essentialaction.org/tobacco/
GLOBALink, The International Tobacco Control Community
  http://www.globalink.org/
  http://gallery.globalink.org
  http://petitions.globalink.org
  http://news.globalink.org English / French / German / Spanish
  news and information
Hamman's research site (Steve Hamann)
  http://hamann.globalink.org/
International Agency on Tobacco and Health (IATH)
  email: admin@iath.org
International Network of Women Against Tobacco (INWAT)
  http://www.inwat.org/
International Network Towards Smoke-Free Hospitals (INTSH)
  http://intsh.globalink.org/
International Non Governmental Coalition Against Tobacco (INGCAT)
  http://www.ingcat.org/
International Society for the Prevention of Tobacco Induced Diseases
  (PTID)
  http://isptid.globalink.org/
International Tobacco Evidence Network (ITEN)
  http://www.tobaccoevidence.net/
Legacy Foundation, tobacco document site
  http://legacy.library.ucsf.edu/cgi/b/bib/bib-idx?g=tob
Corporate Accountabilty International
  www.infact.org
Quit&Win
  http://www.quitandwin.org

Repace Associates, Inc Secondhand Smoke Consultants]
  http://www.repace.com/
Society for Research on Nicotine and Tobacco (SRNT)
  http://www.srnt.org/
Tobaccopedia
  http://TobaccoPedia.org
Tobacco Archives
  http://www.tobaccoarchives.com/
Tobacco BBS (Gene Borio) Tobacco news and information
  http://www.tobacco.org
Tobacco Control journal
  http://www.tobaccocontrol.com
Tobacco Control Archives
  http://www.library.ucsf.edu/tobacco/
Tobacco Control Resource Center/Tobacco Products Liability Project
(TCRC/TPLP)
  http://tobacco.neu.edu/
Tobacco Control Resource Centre (TCRC), BMA, UK
  http://www.tobacco-control.org/
Tobacco Control Supersite (Simon Chapman)
  http://www.health.usyd.edu.au/tobacco/
Tobacco Documents Online (TDO, Smokescreen)
  http://www.tobaccodocuments.org
Treatobacco Database & Educational Resource for Treatment of
  Tobacco Dependence
  http://www.treatobacco.net/
World Conferences on Tobacco or Health
  http://www.wctoh.org

Regional Organizations

European Medical Association on Smoking and Health (EMASH)
  http://emash.globalink.org/
European Network for Smoke-free Hospitals (ENSH)
  http://ensh.free.fr/
European Network for Smoking Prevention (ENSP)
  http://www.ensp.org
European Network of Young People and Tobacco
  http://www.ktl.fi/enypat/
European Network of Quitlines
  http://www.quitlines-conference.com/
Southeast Asia Tobacco Control Alliance
  http://www.tobaccofreeasia.net/

These web and email addresses were accurate in mid-2005. There are,
in addition, many other organizations, wholly or partly working on
tobacco issues, too numerous to include here. These can be contacted
through INGCAT (the International Non Governmental Coalition
Against Tobacco) or FCA. If any would like to be included in future
editions, or on a website, please contact the authors. In addition, we
were unable to include any national and sub-national organizations.

INDEX